The Emperor Needs *New* Clothes

The Emperor Needs *New* Clothes

OR
WHY THE CARING *DISAPPEARED* FROM HEALTH CARE

JEFF WEINBERG, M.ED., M.PH, NHA
NATIONALLY CERTIFIED HEALTH CARE ADVOCATE

Printed in the United States of America.

ISBN: 978-1-63385-473-4

Library of Congress Control Number: 2022919377

Published by:
Word Association Publishers
205 Fifth Avenue
Tarentum, Pennsylvania 15084

www.wordassociation.com
1.800.827.7903

Contents

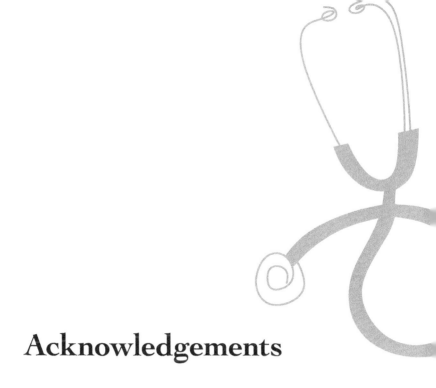

Acknowledgements

There are many people I must thank and recognize for their assistance in helping me write this book.

George Yeckel, PhD., former CEO of Jefferson Hospital, Sister Mulvehill Cresentia, senior vice president of Jefferson Hospital and Sister Paul Gabriel, nursing home consultant. All of them have passed away, however each of them mentored me and helped me become confident in my abilities and successful in the field

1

Ann Gatty, Ph.D.. Owner of Strategic People Solutions. Ann has been my business coach and for the past 9 months we met every couple of weeks to review what I wrote in the book and my progress. Without Ann, I could and would not ever have completed this book. Thank you Ann for all of your assistance.

Friends and colleagues who have contributed their own health care experiences:

Dr. Lisa Mainier, Concierge Physician
and colleague

Ann Llewellyn, RN, One of the leaders in the
field of Health Care Advocacy and colleague

Marla Turnbull, nutritionist and colleague

Former and current caregivers

Lisa Sofko

Dee Bellarby

Peter Gluck, PhD

Marilyn Stollar

Finally a special special thanks to my wife Dee Weinberg, who has been my life partner and has encouraged and supported me in all of my endeavors. I love you all ways!

This book is dedicated to my mother in law, Sarah Mittman Steckel , who died in a nursing home at 97, but she was in perfect health and was there because of multiple falls and balance issues. I used to say, "She doesn't have high blood pressure she gives it!"

She died a tragic and needless death during Covid, due to failure to thrive. She gave up because my wife was no longer able to visit her and her beloved caregivers were unrecognizable in masks and gowns. She also died alone because the administrator had no compassion and would not permit my wife to stay with her in the middle of the night when she was actively dying. Talk about lack of caring!!!

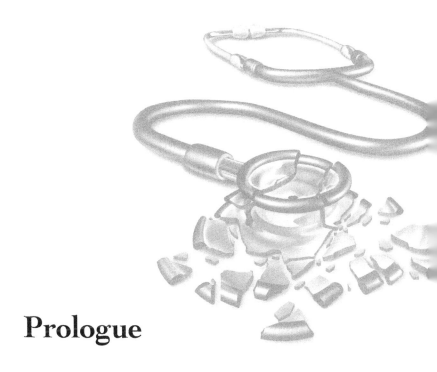

Prologue

In 2020, on the television show, *New Amsterdam*, Dr. Max Goodwin, the chief medical officer, tells a colleague, "When I came here, I wanted to fix this hospital, but now I want to tear it down, to build something better for you, my daughter, and everyone else."

Unfortunately, in this case, fiction does resemble reality. Health care today needs to be torn down to build something better. Health care has become bottom line profit oriented. The caring in health care has largely disappeared. Patients and families are confused about how to navigate the complex medical system. The system has largely taken away the patient's and family's individuality and has taken the caring out of Health Care.

A former client and now friend describes the system as broken:

The System is Broken.

My husband broke his neck in a freak car accident. I never imagined how hard I would have to fight to not only keep him alive, but to get him the care he needed. The system was against us from the beginning. His first day of inpatient rehabilitation, I was grabbed aside and told he had just two weeks there and that I needed to understand how my life was going to change, with round-the-clock care needed for him. How was I going to do this? What was my plan? Why did my husband want to walk again, when there were more important things to focus on? How was I going to do this, did I understand what this means? No, I hadn't even seen my husband yet, but I had to start my training now.

I wanted to just talk with my husband. To work through this with him in my mind…to connect to him and for us to be able to comfort each other.

They told me I could have a cot next to his bed, and I could stay with him every night. But EVERY MINUTE I was there was to be a learning experience, they said. They had to train me every time they made contact with me, they said. I could never just see my husband and talk with him and spend time with him.

He only had two weeks, they said. But I know how this works….every week they submit his progress to insurance and request more time so long as he is making improvements. two weeks, they insisted. And insisted. And I was harassed every minute of every visit with my husband, because I had to learn to care for him, and there's a lot to know. Catheter. Bowel program. Hoyer lift. But wait, he needs more time and I'm going to fight for it! It's based on averages, they told me, and by the way, two people need to learn these things. Who else will be learning? My husband's family came daily but refused to learn care. Every day, I had to learn and by the way, did I ask his family members, who come every day, to get this training because they need two people before he goes home and we only have two weeks. They said no. Nothing I can do. Nobody else will learn. But I need another person and I only have two weeks.

I stayed overnight, craving a night's sleep next to my husband, and a cot was going to have to do. Wake up, you have to turn him. Wake up, time to cath him, wake up, you have to learn this and that and by the way when is someone else going to come in and start learning because two people have to learn this before he can go home in less than two weeks.

I fought like hell through those weeks, and pulled out every stop I could, called in every contact I had in the system, and finally got to a Patient Care Advocate who called a meeting and set things moving in a slightly different direction. My husband got more time in rehab. I got more time with my husband and a checklist of things I could learn at my own pace, instead of being harassed every minute of my visitation time.

This was not perfect, still. Homecoming was imminent, surprising, and poorly coordinated. One day I went in to visit and was told I had a meeting with a doctor who had been looking for me, and he needed to see me ASAP. John was going home. Today.

We had no hospital bed. Did I need one, they asked? We had no wheelchair, they'll lend us one. I had no lift, no medical supplies, nothing.

Amazingly, they came. Quickly. Just before the transport pulled in with my husband, who was sick and depressed, and certainly not ready to leave the hospital environment. Caregivers would eventually come, they said, but not for at least six months, they said. And that was very true, and unfortunate. The red tape is long, and that system is broken as well.

My husband still works part time. I am unable to work, because the system is broken. Caregivers don't show up. Agencies don't have backup. And there is no way to keep a schedule. No amount of fight or Advocacy changes this situation, and there are so many people in the same situation. Couples have to divorce over this, as the abled partner is the one who has to work yet can't do so because of lack of care. You see, the state will pay family members to care for a loved one, EXCEPT spouses. We're just expected to do the care. But if we consider a paper divorce, the state will pay us for round the clock care, you see, until they don't, because we are living there anyway, and well, how many of those hours are you giving care anyway?

And how many benefits does my husband not get, since he is working, that he would get if he was not working? There are so many benefits to get people back to work, but because he works, he is not eligible for them.

Oh my.....the system is broken.

This is very powerful and yet very true. Lisa had to sell her business so she could become a full time caregiver. She now runs a Farm Animal Rescue and continues to be her husband's caregiver with help when she can get it! She is a very brave and remarkable woman.

As a Certified Health Care Patient Advocate, I help patients navigate the complex healthcare system and help them get the individual care they need.

This book discusses how the system operates, or how it is broken, the role of a health care patient advocate, and some suggestions on what to do to change it. It also serves as a primer so people can begin to understand the difference between Medicare, Medicaid, Obama Care, the services available and how they are paid for, and how to better navigate the system.

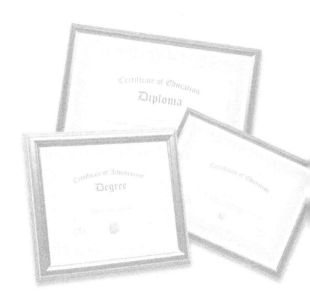

My Background in Health Care

I have been in health care for over 25 years. Since I first started, the landscape of health care has changed drastically. It has moved away from emphasizing personal health care and well-being care and transformed into a profit driven model controlled by insurance and pharmaceutical companies.

I began my career working in mental health as a clinician and director of outpatient MH/MR/D&A. I had earned a master's degree in Counselor Education from Duquesne University. At that time, 1963, President John F. Kennedy initiated Community Mental Health Services because of his sister being institutionalized when Kennedy was a child.

Here is what President Kennedy said: "I am proposing a new approach to mental illness and to mental retardation. This approach is designed, in large measure, to use Federal resources to stimulate state, local and private action. When carried out, reliance on the cold mercy of custodial isolation will be supplanted by the open warmth of community concern and capability. Emphasis on prevention, treatment and rehabilitation will be substituted for a desultory interest in confining patients in an institution to wither away." — *John F. Kennedy, Special Message to the Congress on Mental Illness and Mental Retardation, February 5, 1963*

The bill that President Kennedy passed reversed 100 years of non-involvement by the Federal government. As a result of the Kennedy bill, numerous outpatient mental health centers were developed throughout the country. The outpatient center where I worked provided a complete continuum of care. This included an acute inpatient hospital and three outpatient mental health centers of which I supervised two of them, and a comprehensive drug and alcohol program.

In addition, the center had a day and night partial hospitalization program. We developed one of the first Employee Assistance Programs with United States Steel Corporation and the City of Pittsburgh employees.

I also oversaw the development of a social service program with the Graduate School of Social Work at the University of Pittsburgh. This program was created for low-income residents in apartments in the community. The program included weekly health screenings and a graduate social work student available to help residents who needed someone to talk through challenges they were experiencing.

This initiative eventually became the beginning of our Area on Aging programs. I was one of the founding board members. Also, it is important to note that this program was established as a reimbursement program but was considered community outreach prevention.

Another program which I initiated under community outreach prevention was called **C.O.P.E.**

(Children's Onsite Psychiatric and Education Program). This was geared toward acting out adolescents in the schools. They would come to our center twice a week in the afternoon for group therapy, community activities and outings. This was under the supervision of a child psychiatrist who was employed by our facility.

I remember one Easter when this group wanted to distribute candy to disabled children who were living in a facility. This had a profound effect on the group members. They always felt their problems were the worst. Many of them came from single parent homes with many parents battling drug or alcohol addiction or who were rarely home. After the Easter candy visit, group members realized their problems were not as bad as they thought. They started to stop acting out and started to concentrate on how they could make their lives better. One member later became a juvenile probation officer.

The outpatient mental health center developed many outreach and prevention programs, which included a program to deal with high-risk pregnant mothers to prevent failure to thrive babies.

I can remember the director of prevention services saying that their programs could reach more people than any counseling or therapy program.

However, this direct funding stream went away in the early 80s when President Reagan eliminated federal funding for mental health services and created Block Grant Funding which allowed the states to determine how they were going to spend the Federal money given to them. Today mental health services are still not funded with any federal government monies. Yet, the need for these services has never been greater due to gun violence, the Pandemic and social isolation, and business closings and unemployment skyrocketing.

When Federal funding stopped, the center formed one outpatient mental health center where all the directors took a 10% pay cut and our salaries were frozen. The center went from 140 professionals to 10.

All of us were the most senior in the system. This is when I sought my additional academic degree. I obtained a master's degree in Public Health Administration (M.PH) at the University of Pittsburgh and specialized in Geriatric Services.

At the time, I should have realized that funding will always be a central issue. To this day, mental health services are largely unfunded, so people cannot afford the medical help or medication they need. In other words, our fellow citizens go without the essential mental health services that could provide life-altering assistance.

After obtaining my M.PH degree, I became a licensed nursing home administrator in Pennsylvania and in Florida. At one point I worked for a major health system as director of senior services. I was asked to be chair of a committee within the organization, charged with examining the delivery of health care to seniors. We were to analyze both internal and external care. The committee was comprised of senior management, department heads and community members at large. The committee was under the direction of the Senior Vice President of the Health Center, Sr Crescentia Mulvihill. She was also one of my mentors and I am deeply grateful for the positive influence she had on my career

Internally, we looked at senior services and found them to be fragmented, with each department operating in a silo. There was no continuity of care! We also looked at our furniture and signage and found that we were not very senior friendly.

Externally, we found that there was little emphasis on prevention, and the community was unable to access care because no transportation was available. In addition, there was no follow up after the patient was discharged.

Based on our findings the committee developed a plan to address these needs. My responsibility was to report our findings and recommendations to the Foundation Board. This was the group of people who ultimately would fund this project. However, Senior Management was split on whether to pursue the plan because they did not believe it generated revenue. I told some of the officers that the system was turning down "Motherhood, Apple Pie, Hot dogs, and Chevrolet!" (A common expression at the time.) Alas, we did get some of what we proposed, but it was a hybrid that would not have the impact we deemed necessary.

From there the system got worse. First the Health System President, George Yeckel, CEO, another mentor, was forced to step down. Then, my supervisor, Senior Vice President Sister Crescentia also was forced to retire. The new appointed president was a bank officer. The focus of the health system changed to making organizational decisions based solely on profit margin.

This philosophy was out of alignment with everything I believed about senior health care. It was time to depart. I found a new home with the Pittsburgh Jewish Association on Aging. As their first Vice President, I was responsible for developing aging services for the resident Jewish

Community, as well as designing methods for improving the care we could provide. Things seemed to be promising here and I felt I would be able to help contribute to my Jewish Community.

The Jewish Association on Aging staff needed training on customer service, teamwork, working with people with dementia, and taking pride in what they did. During my tenure, I noticed troubling patterns. There were many staff call offs which directly affected patient care. This was difficult to address because the staff had a union that protected them. I wanted to increase our staffing numbers so that we would have enough staff to provide quality care despite call-offs. The person I reported to, the president of the JAA, continually reiterated that I was not focused enough on budgeting. I knew that if we provided quality care our census would be full, our employees would be proud of their work, and it would improve care. Instead, they were stressed, overworked, and felt unappreciated. I started a program called Pride in Care with the University of Pittsburgh, Graduate School of Social Work. Each employee was trained in customer service and taking pride in their work.

Ultimately, the facility began to provide better care and we had the best annual survey from the Department of Health in about 7 years.

While we were working on improving care, I initiated a dementia program and a behavioral health program with Western Psychiatric Institute. The goal was to prevent rehospitalization for residents who continued to exhibit external behavior issues. Lastly, I built in collaboration with the University of Pittsburgh Dental School a dental office in the facility to provide free dental care to our residents.

Finally, plans were in place to build a new assistive living facility in the heart of the community as well as downsizing and building a new nursing home from 300 beds to a 120-bed facility, each having private rooms.

As all of this was going on, we began to remodel the 300-bed facility starting with the lobby and common areas. However, the president of the JAA did not want residents sitting in the lobby, because it would detract from the appearance of the lobby. As I was leaving, he changed the management of our food service department which was dedicated to serving quality kosher food to another vendor which provided less staffing and a lower quality kosher food.

This is when I developed the idea for writing this book. In reality, *The Emperor Needs New Clothes*. Patient health care was being provided based on "mirrors." By this I mean that if the facility appeared nice and clean, then this demonstrates that the care must be good as well.

Throughout my career, this concept continues to be reinforced. Make facilities appear to have all the finest amenities and mask the less than adequate care. This is scary. More individuals are entering these facilities without understanding what is occurring daily.

Our acute and long-term health care delivery system is severely broken. It needs to be rebuilt from the ground floor. It is important that anyone who may need these services is aware of how to discern what is out there. This is not an industry that should be solely guided by financial reports, profit and loss statements and profit margins. It is time to reverse this trend and show respect for our elder population and provide quality care that is available.

This book will address these issues, as well as discuss the need for health care patient advocates and present recommended solutions to many of these challenges.

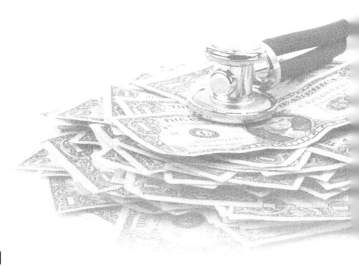

CHAPTER 1

How We Got Here

To understand why health care has become profit-oriented and insurance-driven, we must look at the history of what became a health care industry. Secondly, we must examine the whole structure of financial reimbursement as established by the health insurance industry.

When Europeans colonized North America in the 1600s, they brought the concept of almshouses with them. When someone couldn't be taken care of by family or neighbor, then they were put into an institution that was largely run by the county, village, or other government entity, explains Harvard geriatrician, professor, and scholar Muriel R. Gilllick. She authored the 2018 book, *Old and Sick in America: the Journey through the Health Care System*. Almshouses housed not only elderly, but also orphans, people with disabilities, those facing addiction and the homeless. Almshouses provided shelter and meals only. The almshouses evolved into old age homes. These were largely run by religious and ethnic organizations that felt it was their mission to care for these members of their own culture.

Throughout this book I track the Jewish Home for the Aged in Pittsburgh along with other religious and government operated homes. I also include descriptions of for-profit facilities located throughout Western Pennsylvania.

The Jewish Home for the Aged or Beth Moshab Z'Kenim [House for the Settlement of the Elderly] was dedicated in 1906. It was founded in response to the perceived need for kosher housing for the elderly by Rabbi Aaron Mordecai Ashinsky. The charter, dated January 19, 1906, stated its mission as "maintaining a home or house for aged Hebrews in conformity with ...Orthodox Judaism." Money was collected throughout western Pennsylvania,

West Virginia, and eastern Ohio with the understanding that the Home would accept elderly Jews from the tri-state region.

In 1933, the Home added a new building on 17 acres of land in Squirrel Hill. The Jewish Association on Aging, formed in 1993, and located on that site, now administers a comprehensive continuum of care of services and facilities that support older adults.

I became the first Vice President of the Jewish Association on Aging and was responsible for running a 300+ bed nursing home facility as well as planning new services for the community. As stated earlier, I started my career as a nursing home administrator there 10 years prior. I had just finished my master's degree at the University of Pittsburgh, Graduate School of Public Health and needed a 6-month internship working with a licensed nursing home administrator. Upon completion, I was able to sit for the exam and become a licensed nursing home administrator.

During this period, the Jewish Home for the Aged changed its name to Riverview Center for Jewish Seniors. It was moving away from taking care of the poor under a benevolent care program and moving to a medical model where residents needed assistance with nursing care and rehabilitation. This was largely funded by private pay, insurances, Medicare, and Medicaid.

In the 1946 Congress passed the Hill Burton Act, which changed the focus of facilities housing older people. Now the focus would become centered on providing medical care. These facilities looked and were modeled after hospitals. In addition to the model of nursing homes changing from benevolent housing to medical care, third party reimbursement changed and continues to change. The adage "Follow the Money" is truer than ever! Nursing homes were embracing the same profit motivation as hospitals were now embracing.

In 1935, the Social Security Act was implemented. This was the period during the 1930s Great Depression. At that time 50% of the elderly were indigent. President Franklin D. Roosevelt signed the new act, creating a social insurance program designed to pay retired workers, age 65 or older, income after retirement.

In 1965 Title XVIII and Title XIX were passed. This provided health insurance coverage for people who were on Social Security and were disabled. (Medicare) Title XIX provided health insurance coverage for those who were indigent. (Medicaid)

Now this gets tricky, pay attention!

Hospitals and nursing homes were paid based on **retrospective reimbursement system**. This meant that the cost of care was billed as charges not actual costs. People used to complain that the cost of an aspirin in the hospital was between 6 and 10 dollars. While the actual cost of the aspirin is pennies! The hospital would add on the cost of the pharmacist to dispense it, label it, and the nurse to administer it. In addition, there was no requirement for discharge until the doctor decided to discharge.

In 1965 my mother had a heart attack and was in the hospital for almost 2 months. Today that same person would be in the hospital 4 days unless there were complications.

My daughter had her first child 15 years ago in 2006 and she was in the hospital for 5 days and they had a steak dinner compliment of the hospital. When her second child was born 3 years after, they sent her home after one night stay with a package of peanut butter crackers! So, what has changed?

Reimbursement changed from **retroactive to prospective**. This meant that hospitals could no longer bill on a cost to charges ratio but on just cost of service.

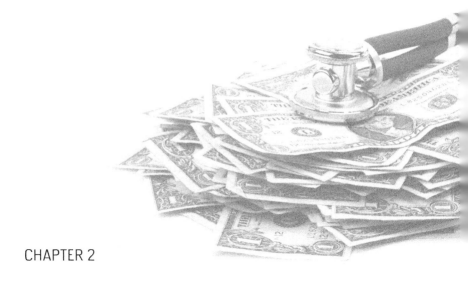

CHAPTER 2

Prospective Reimbursement

Around 1985, Medicare and other insurances developed a prospective payment system of reimbursement called DRGs (Diagnostic Related Groupings), the average cost based on 467 diagnostic/ reimbursement categories. These diagnoses were converted to a total cost for care and length of stay for discharge. The length of stay varied based on severity of the diagnoses.

Let's take a look what this means. For someone diagnosed with pneumonia, the average length of stay was determined at 5.2 days according to the DRG, and Medicare would reimburse about $10,000. This amount was all inclusive, meaning staffing, medications, supplies, and tests were part of the lump sum paid to the hospital. If someone was discharged in 4 days the hospital would get reimbursed $10,000. If the person was discharged in 6 days the hospital would still get paid $10,000.

So the incentive was to discharge earlier than the length of stay. Another incentive was to reduce the number of tests ordered in order to reduce costs. Today your primary physician rarely admits patients or makes rounds in the hospital. The hospitals have physicians called hospitalists. These physicians are salaried hospital employees and follow the hospital protocols for the number of tests ordered and length of stay. Hospitals start the discharge process on admission and now discharge patients sicker and sooner!

As a health care patient advocate, I am called many times by a family member saying their loved one is being discharged to a nursing home tomorrow and they don't think they are ready for discharge and don't know what nursing home to pick. If they are not ready for discharge, I intervene so they can stay longer or find an alternative place for discharge instead of nursing homes. During Covid, a client's wife had multiple organ failures. The case manager wanted to discharge her to a nursing home.

I recommended a LTAC (Long Term Acute Care Hospital), where she would receive more care and also the family was permitted to visit because it was a hospital and not a nursing home, where families were not permitted to visit during Covid. (More about this later.)

Sometimes, clients can benefit from acute rehabilitation hospitals where staffing provided more care and the person received extensive therapy 3 hours per day. People who have a stroke, multiple fractures, spinal cord injuries can benefit from more extensive therapy.

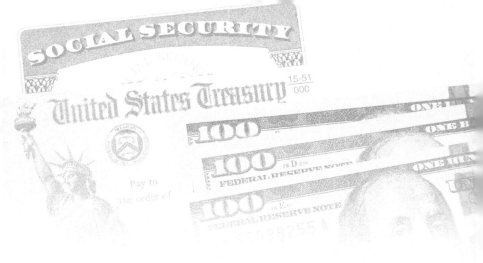

CHAPTER 3

Understanding Medicare and Medicaid Insurances

As discussed before, Medicare and Medicaid legislation was passed by the US Congress and signed into law by President Johnson in 1965 as Title XVIII and Title XIX. Medicare provided health insurance for everyone that had worked when they reached the age of 65 or were disabled. Medicaid was made available for anyone who was at poverty level and could not afford health care. There is much confusion about what medical expenses Medicare covers as well as Medicaid. We'll start by explaining the major parts of Medicare Insurance that are provided through the government and then describe the Medicare Advantage Health Insurance that is a program provided through private health insurance companies.

Medicare coverage is based on 3 main factors:

1. Federal and state laws.
2. National coverage decisions made by Medicare about whether something is covered.
3. Local coverage decisions made by companies in each state that process claims for Medicare. These companies decide whether something is medically necessary and should be covered in their area.

The government Medicare program includes Medicare Part A (hospital insurance) and Part B (medical insurance). If you want drug coverage, you can join a separate Medicare drug plan (Part D). You can use any doctor or hospital that takes the government Medicare, anywhere in the U.S.

Medicare Part A Premium

Under Part A hospital in-patient related costs are covered. There are several aspects to be tracking.

1. **Be aware of the difference between observation days and acute in-patient status.** However, if someone is admitted for OBSERVATION DAYS, Medicare only pays for part of the stay because it is not considered an acute hospital admission. Observation status used to be if one presents themselves to the emergency room and the hospital staff was undecided about whether to admit them or whether to send them home. So, the hospital staff would admit the individual for 23 hours. If the symptoms get worse, they would admit the patient to acute in-patient care, if not they would send them home.

I want you to know that a hospital can admit a person to in-patient acute care for as many days as they want and the patient is not aware of this. The notice of observation status is part of several papers given to the patient.

As a health care patient advocate, I have come across this situation numerous times. The patient needs to be given INFORMED CONSENT, which means the information is reviewed and understood by the patient and acknowledged by signing the document. On one occasion, a client who was very ill was in the hospital and the family became aware that he was on observation status. I was told that the physician had to change the status. When I questioned the physician, he thought the patient was on in-patient status all along, so after I informed the physician, he changed the status retroactively back to the date of admission. Physicians are rarely aware of the admission status, nor are they informed. This status is determined by a case manager.

The reason observation status changed from 23 hours to as many days as deemed necessary (are you ready for this?). Medicare now penalizes hospitals for readmitting someone prior to 30 days of discharge. Observation days are not counted, so hospitals are not penalized for readmitting patients within 30 days because the patient was technically never admitted to the acute in patient stay to start off with.

2. Medicare Part A also covers acute in-patient rehabilitation. This is an alternative to Skilled Nursing Rehabilitation. Usually, one must be able to tolerate 3 hours of therapy per day. This is a combination of physical, occupational and speech therapies. Patients get about 1.5 hours in the morning and 1.5 hours in the afternoon. Patients must have a medical necessity as well, such as a stroke, spinal cord injury, multiple fractures, or a brain injury. The rehab team is supervised by a rehab doctor called a Physiatrist. The Physiatrist rounds daily with the rehab team and sees each patient. Unfortunately, this alternative is rarely brought up by a discharge social worker.

This occurred in the health system I worked in. We developed a state-of-the-art rehab program with a car on the unit, mini store for shopping, a bank machine, a kitchen, and a real bedroom with a bed instead of a hospital bed. I will never forget when we first developed this and had a patient sleep in the room with his wife, we were told that this was the first time he slept with his wife in 10 years. All of these were developed so that the patient can be prepared for home. The concept is called a Therapeutic Milleu where therapy in the gym is duplicated and practiced on the unit. Unfortunately, the social workers in the hospital would not discharge to us and this has continued to the present!

As a health care advocate, I have stopped several patients going to a skilled nursing facility and have gotten them into an acute rehab center. Discharge social workers want to get the patients out of the hospital as quick as possible, where skilled nursing facilities will take patients sight unseen, acute rehab has to evaluate the person face to face. This extra day in the hospital prevents the patient from benefiting from the more extensive service because they usually must stay an extra day and it will cost the hospital money by keeping them longer.

3. Part A Medicare does pay for skilled nursing and rehabilitation stay. The coverage for the first 20 days is paid in full, then they pay 80% from days 21 – 100. The patient pays the 20%. or approximately $197.50 per day. This is usually covered by a secondary insurance such as AARP. If the patient does not have a secondary insurance, they have to pay this fee privately or apply for Medicaid, which you need to prove that your income is at poverty level.

4. Another area covered by Part A is called home health care. People must be homebound after a hospitalization or stay in a nursing or rehab facility and need extended skilled nursing care in the home. Skilled nursing is defined as nursing by a licensed nurse and or continued therapy. These professionals usually visit about 3 times a week until the service is no longer needed. However, most people get confused between Home Health

Care and Home Care. Home care is attendant care where someone is hired to assist with activities of daily living (i.e. Bathing, dressing, toileting, eating, transferring, and walking). Home Care is NOT covered by Medicare or health insurance. One must pay privately for these services which cost about $25. 00/HR.

If someone has long term care insurance, home care is covered. If a spouse or patient served in the Armed Forces during a wartime, they might be eligible for payment for home care under Aid and Attendance Program. Call the Veteran's Administration or an elder law attorney to learn about eligibility. Low-income families may qualify for a waiver program through their County Area on Aging.

5. Another unknown service that Part A covers is an LTACH (Long Term Acute Care Hospital). These are facilities that specialize in the treatment of patients with serious medical conditions that require care on an ongoing basis but no longer require intensive care or extensive diagnostic procedures. These patients are typically discharged from the intensive care units and require more care than they can receive in a rehabilitation center, skilled nursing facility, or at home. The average length of stay is about 30 days. Once again, social workers in the hospital rarely refer patients to LTACH .

.Instead, they are referred to nursing homes.

As a health care patient advocate, I have often had patients go to an LTACH so that they can get stabilized before they return home. Health Care Patient Advocates provide family members with alternatives to care so that the family members can make intelligent decisions.

6. Last, Part A pays for Hospice Care. This is usually End of Life Care. The patient has less than 6 months to live due to a terminal illness or a condition where there was no hope of someone's health would get better. Comfort Care is provided such as pain management, but usually the patient does not return to that hospital for other conditions and treatments, such as resuscitation, tube feedings and ventilators.

As a health care advocate, I always check for an Advanced Directive or Living Will. This is a legal document that designates what the patient wants at end of life and designates someone to fulfill those wishes if the patient cannot express these wishes. Also, the advanced directive designates a financial power of attorney to manage the patient's money when they are unable to do so themselves. Everyone should have these important documents as they age.

Medicare Part B Premium

This government funded insurance covers 2 types of services:

1. *Medically necessary services:* Services or supplies that are needed to diagnose or treat your medical condition and that meet accepted standards of medical practice.

2. *Preventive services:* Health care to prevent illness (like the flu) or detect it at an early stage when treatment is most likely to work.

Part B coverage is generally considered outpatient care. This includes:

- Physician services
- Lab, X rays, Blood Work
- Medical Equipment and Supplies
- Orthotics and Prosthetics
- Mental Health Care
- Ambulance Services

Unfortunately, Part B does NOT cover vision exams and eyeglasses, hearing exams and hearing aids, dental exams and dentures, implants, or treatments. As we age, we naturally decline in these areas. Yet because of lack of financial assistance most seniors cannot afford hearing aids, glasses, or dentures.

No one realizes that not receiving proper medical assistance in these three areas has consequences. Hearing loss causes cognitive issues, anxiety, depression, and other mental health issues. Vision loss causes similar symptoms. Dental issues can cause swallowing and choking issues, leading to pneumonia and poor nutrition.

The Part B Premium of $148.50 is taken out of your monthly social security. This premium increases annually. Individuals should sign up for Part B when they reach the age of 65. It is important to note that if someone does not sign up and arrange for monthly payments they can be fined and penalized.

Medicare Advantage Plan, Part C.

Part C is often called Managed Medicare; however, it is really managed cost. I refer to this plan as a Medicare Disadvantage Plan!

It is offered by private health insurance companies approved by Medicare. Medicare Advantage Plans are all inclusive covering hospital (all Part A services), outpatient and physician (all Part B services) and a prescription drug plan (Part D coverage). On the surface it appears that Part C is truly an advantage plan because it is all inclusive. Some of the more expensive plans cover vision, dental and hearing.

HOWEVER, your choice is limited to hospitals, physicians, pharmacies that have a contract with that insurance company. The insurance company contracts with facilities and physicians which contain costs. Also, if you need health care coverage in an area outside where you live, the only service that would be covered is the visit and care in a hospital emergency room. Everything else is paid for out of pocket unless you opt out of the Part C program and utilize Medicare coverage.

Medicare provides coverage no matter where you are in the country. For example, if someone lives in the north and usually goes south for the winter, the only way to be covered is with Medicare. From October through December you are able to opt out of the plan you are enrolled in annually and change coverage.

IT IS VITALLY IMPORTANT
That You Consult A Health Insurance Expert Who Sells All Health Insurance Policies.

This consultation is free to you. Your insurance agent gets paid by the company based on renewals and meets with you annually as your circumstances may have changed or there is   a better product for you the following year.

Medicare Part D

Medicare Part D covers prescription drugs. You can enroll in a prescription plan through a private company. Reminder, if you are enrolled in Part C, Medicare Advantage plan you are already covered for prescription drugs.

It is important to review a plan's formulary, which is a list of covered prescriptions, to ensure that you can get the medicine you need without paying for it out of pocket. If you log in to Medicare.gov/plan- compare Medicare will help you pick your best option by completing your drug formulary.

I helped a friend and his wife save about $1000 a month by having him talk with a health insurance provider.

AGAIN, IT IS VITALLY IMPORTANT THAT YOU CONSULT A HEALTH INSURANCE EXPERT WHO SELLS ALL POLICIES, so that you get the coverage you need or want.

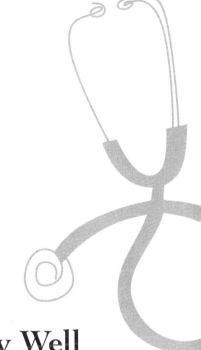

CHAPTER 4

They Don't Play Well in the Sandbox!

In Pittsburgh, we have two major health systems: University of Pittsburgh Medical Center (UPMC) and Allegheny Health Network (AHN)

On the UPMC website, it is reported that the first quarter 2021, UPMC operating income grew 9% to 288 million dollars. On the same website, UPMC is described as a 23-billion-dollar provider and insurer. UPMC owns 34 hospitals in Pennsylvania, and Western New York, and one hospital in Maryland.

But it doesn't stop there. UPMC owns or partners with hospitals in Italy, China, Kazakatan, and Ireland, yet with 23 billion dollars in their treasure chest, they are a not-for-profit corporation so they do not pay taxes.

Now don't get me wrong, UPMC is a world class health system ranked in the top 15 health systems in the country, with excellent physicians, equipment, and care. They have made a lot of money and yet many consumers cannot access or afford the care they need.

The saying "follow the money" has been truer than ever. Former UPMC CEO, Jeffrey Romoff, who recently retired, made 9.5 million dollars in salary and benefits. A number of years ago the company bought the former US Steel building in downtown Pittsburgh, which is also the tallest building in the city, and added a 20-foot sign on top of the building.

Allegheny Health Network which is owned by Highmark Insurance (Blue Cross/Blue Shield) is UPMC's major competitor. Allegheny Health Network (AHN), based in Pittsburgh, is a non-profit, 13-hospital academic medical system with facilities located in Western Pennsylvania and one hospital in Western New York. AHN was formed in 2013 when Highmark Inc., a

Pennsylvania-based Blue Cross Blue Shield insurance carrier, purchased the assets of the West Penn Allegheny Health System (WPAHS) and added three more hospitals to its provider division. Allegheny Health Network was formed to act as the parent company to the WPAHS hospitals and its affiliate hospitals. Highmark Health today serves as the ultimate parent of AHN.

Allegheny General is their flagship Hospital. Their revenue reported in 2020 was 3.65 billion dollars compared to UPMC's 23 billion dollars. AHN operating income in 2020 was 169 million dollars compared to UPMC's 288 million dollars in the first quarter of 2021. Both have similar services and are world-renowned. However, many enrollees do not have access to services and doctors if they are insured by UPMC or Highmark. Cancer patients were permitted to access both Systems, but UPMC started to deny cancer patients with other insurances.

In an article by Kris Mamula of the *Pittsburgh Post-Gazette* on April 19, 2019, a woman was denied access to her UPMC physician she had been seeing because she had Highmark insurance.

Her doctor at UPMC Hillman Cancer Center in Shadyside found a new drug to try. It worked, easing her night sweats, fatigue, and nausea. Now, the challenges of her treatment were being complicated by RULES rather than medical decisions. This case and many others led to the Pa. Attorney General suing UPMC.

Pennsylvania Attorney General Josh Shapiro sued in 2019 to keep health giant UPMC from ending its business relationship with rival Highmark Health, so that patients could continue care with their treating physicians and in hopes of preventing higher costs from hitting about 70,000 western Pennsylvania patients. The attorney general's office wanted the court to impose a single, modified consent decree that would continue the business relationship between UPMC and Highmark, both based in Pittsburgh, two of Pennsylvania's largest charitable institutions. Highmark had agreed to Shapiro's proposed deal, but UPMC had not.

The key issue is that both companies are not for profit charitable institutions which should provide access to any service regardless of coverage or inability to pay.

Shapiro is quoted as saying, "UPMC has not been living up to its obligations as a public charity, a status that gives it protection from taxes. The attorney general's petition accused UPMC of wasting charitable assets through "exorbitant executive salaries and perquisites in the form of corporate jets and prestigious office space waste."

Just recently UPMC, was sued by the Federal Government alleging civil fraud (Pittsburgh Business Times, September 10-16, 2021).

The suit claims that since 2015 (or possibly earlier), Dr. Luketich, Chair of the UPMC Department of Cardiothoracic surgery, performed 3 surgeries at the same time. He was simultaneously working back and forth between 3 operating rooms. The suit alleges that he left surgical patients unattended for hours at a time. He falsely attested that he was with these patients throughout the entirety of the surgery. He unlawfully billed the government health benefit programs for these procedures. This activity was to increase surgical volume, maximize UPMC revenue. and/or appease Luketich. Talk about greed and depersonalization.

As one can see, these rivalries do not play well in the sandbox. Instead of allowing the consumer to decide where and when they want to see a certain doctor or go to a certain specialty hospital, the providers prevent them from making these choices. Once again Medicare Advantage (Part C) is Medicare Disadvantage and Managed Care becomes Managed Costs.

Dr. Lisa Manier. a colleague, discusses this further from a physician perspective:

What does a girl who has always been enchanted with bugs under a microscope do for a living? She may become a scientist. In this case, she becomes a physician.

There once was a young girl who explored nature in the smallest of ways. She read books about small bugs, bacteria, viruses, cells, plants, seeds and more. A fabulous summer day consisted of pulling water from her "grass clipping stew" to view under her microscope, all kinds of creatures growing in the brew. She grew up. She studied anatomy, physiology, biochemistry, and embryology in college. How could one live in her own body without knowing and appreciating such marvel? The human body and its function are truly astonishing. How could discovery stop there?

This girl studied all kinds of cells and tissues, how they formed, changed, and managed to become diseased and aberrant. This intrigued her as she grew into her career in pathology. She continued to study disease from a molecular, cellular, and eventually, a clinical perspective, as she entered clinical medicine as a physician assistant. The thrill was on. As she delved into orthopedic surgery, gross tissue, anatomy, function, and malfunction, all began to make sense in an even larger way.

My name is Dr. Lisa Mainier. My medical career began long before medical school. In fact, medical school, residency, and fellowship were the later steps to where I now find myself. The most exciting toy under the Christmas tree was a microscope left to me by Santa at the age of eight! I could not wait until summer to "brew" microorganisms and drop them on the slide to see what was growing in nature's tea. My most exciting science class was in fifth grade when my science teacher introduced a different body system each Friday morning. I found the workings of the body wondrous. . . and I still do. I started my career in pathology after graduation from college. My first exposure to "medicine" began at the cellular level. I understood how disease and changes occur from a cellular, biochemical and molecular level, long before diving into the depths of clinical and surgical medicine. My goal was to eventually become a forensic pathologist, just like "Quincy"! (A former television program about a medical examiner starring Jack Klugman in the late 70s) Unfortunately, the medical career in pathology never came to fruition, but my love for the true, scientific and foundational view of medicine never got lost in the acculturation of the clinical, medical and surgical context.

My education in health care administration and risk management, although not one of my favorite deviations, certainly added to the gestalt view of medicine as I developed into the clinical realm. It allowed me a "peek" into how medical care was driven.

I wanted to apply what I knew to actually make a difference in people's lives. Eventually, I became a physician. I enjoyed studying medicine. I felt grateful to be able to study deeply, everything and anything regarding how the human body worked and how it became "diseased".

I chose to become an osteopathic physician. In addition to the medical curriculum, I was able to learn medicine from a structural and holistic point of view, which I believed would arm me with a greater depth of knowledge to aid in healing.

You can imagine my surprise when I began my internship after medical school. The clinical focus was on collecting just enough history from the patient in order to make a diagnosis based on an ICD, or diagnosis code. The purpose of the code? To lead me to appropriate studies and treatments which usually consisted of medication and or therapies that may or may not have helped the patient and usually required persistent follow up and monitoring. In many cases, the therapy caused different symptoms, which was considered an "acceptable" collateral consequence.

The emphasis of treatment for patient chronic conditions concentrated on long term treatments to forestall worsening symptoms, but rarely to eliminate the conditions in the first place. There was always an underlying theory that family history, genetics and age was at the root issue of chronic disease and was considered an unavoidable process. In medicine, prevention consists of "catching it early" with screening programs. These are designed to find a disease after the process has begun in a theoretical effort to "treat early" to thwart more serious disease.

Very rarely in my training, did I ever witness a meaningful conversation with a patient regarding environmental factors, nutritional intake, or activity level as a serious and effective part of prevention or treatment.

Perhaps a brief comment "you have to lose weight" may have been uttered, confusing for most and frustrating for the rest. Nutrition, activity level and personal environment is rarely if ever, discussed with patients. Some practitioners and physicians fail to display personal attention to healthy lifestyle habits which can also send confusing messages.

When I began medical school, I was not completely sure where to go with medicine, but I knew I had a penchant and talent for orthopedics and surgery. I wished to retain my surgical skills. As students and residents, we decide (decide what?) based on rotations during medical school and internship. Students, interns, and residents "see" a lot during various rotations. For some observers, the politics and mores register and are taken into consideration during the decision-making process. Predictions may be made about a particular specialty in medicine, which aids in the decision process. For instance, when I was rotating with a urogynecologist, I noted her logging RVUs, or Relative Value Units, most of the clinical time, between and after patients. She also shared a letter sent by administrators that she was not "keeping up" with surgeries. In short, she was "letting patients go" without booking them for surgery. I quickly realized that as a surgeon, she was viewed as a high-volume technician in the operating room for the medical system, not a talented physician who should be making decisions based on individual patient need or medical care. Her "value" to the large hospital system that employed her had not to do with patient healing, quality of life and healthful outcomes, it had to do with profit.

That and many other scenarios during my internship deflated my goal to continue in a specialty. Many surgeons were being driven to produce, were not seen as professionals or experts to guide patients to healthful lives. From my perspective, specialists were seen as profit-drivers and machines. I am not sure the surgeons realized or cared how they were viewed. I witnessed some of my classmates struggling through residencies, fellowships and sub fellowships only to be driven hard to produce profit for large hospital systems that had them jumping from office to office, working long hours in services unrelated to patient care and denied the ability to develop a relationship with their patients a truly healing process.

I was asked to join a family medicine residency program during my internship. That was not my goal or desire, but it would allow me to consider medicine in a general manner and then decide how to continue from there. During residency, I continued to endure the "indoctrination" of incorporating pre-determined, inflexible, protocols and algorithms as patient care. Those protocols were designed to allow various levels of medical staff to dole out the same "expertise" to the patients without much understanding. A one-size-fits-all approach – which is easier to implement, assures standardization and is lower in cost - is what drives many specialties and does not take into consideration patient quality of life or even the attainment of health.

I found the current practice of medicine unchallenging, meaningless, and incomplete. It appeared to be intentionally designed to make the patient dependent on an unrelenting, cyclic dependence on care.

Once graduating from residency, I secured a position in occupational medicine, consisting of a great deal of musculoskeletal injuries and orthopedics. I was elated to be back in the game. Although I loved the concentration in injury medicine, I quickly began to realize that this kind of medicine while challenging and exciting, very rapidly felt like assembly line medical care. The time that I used to spend teaching patients was not permitted in the very strict time constraints. The word "doctor" translates to "teacher", and this is where most providers are lacking in ability and drive. In the past, I have been able to explain injuries and the healing process to patients in terms that they could very easily understand. This allowed the development of relationships and a sense of trust in me as a physician, which endorsed patient participation and control in the healing process.

The work experience left me feeling deeply dissatisfied and morally compromised. I had allowed my integrity and professionalism to become violated. Pushing patients through, denying my drive to practice professionally, abandoning my values and principles to meet ever-increasing quotas, felt wrong. Over time, I felt more like chattel whose job was to produce profit for some money-hungry autocracy, rather than be an expert in healing. Personally, I felt exhausted, unhealthy, frustrated and my professional standing as a physician, withered.

I believed I would not only lose the ability to give patients what they really wanted and what I had to offer but realized that my talent was not a valued commodity in the medical system that exists today. It is now a system that is driven by profit, reduced overhead, treatment instead of healing, and the demand for the illusion of patient satisfaction.

I experienced strong conflicts with my work and maintaining professional integrity. I was embarrassed to finally realize that this is the medicine for which I was being prepared in medical school and residency. It all became quite clear that the process would not improve but would most likely worsen. I loved working with my co-workers, the patients, the overall challenge of the job and the cases. I was so conflicted, but things had to change. My self-worth became more important than monetary gain. I had a choice to neglect my value system and collect a paycheck or begin practicing on my own.

The risk of starting a private practice would be an uphill, lonely, and difficult journey. I felt that my fellow physicians viewed my decision as "throwing in the towel" when in reality, I was really quite brave. I am one of the few fearless physicians to endure on her own.

I chose to avoid the unethical political arena that exists in medicine today. I chose to avoid physician "employers" and insurance company demands. I chose to use my experience, extensive and varied education, common sense, insight, well-honed cognitive abilities, to practice medicine in a meaningful way. No one dictates my time when it comes to patient care. Much like a lawyer, architect, CPA and other professional service providers, I charge a fee for my time and expertise. I am one of the few physicians who realize that I have a right to use my talent, education, and experience to make an honorable, yet prosperous living.

I work in my own thriving preventive medicine practice. I see a few patients each day, spending sufficient time to hear their stories, in which are embedded various clues associated with their concerns. Patients report feeling more like a person and less like broken objects in my office. They report a sense of being taken seriously, not judged. They are surprised when they are given feasible recommendations that facilitate healing and improved well-being. An approachable, competent, and understanding physician is what they find. This is in direct opposition to the mammoth medical systems whose employed providers efficiently populate an electronic medical record with virtually incomplete and often inaccurate history for the purposes of fulfilling data requirements. I am not limited by the Electronic Medical Record "pre-written" history, time constraints and over-reaching inexperienced administrators, accountants, and non-practicing physicians.

There is no insurance company, accountant or administrator running the medical show in my practice. What happens in my practice *stays* in my practice. The patient's history is for assessment, not for reimbursement. All reported, collected or offered information is for the benefit of the patient's evaluation, not for insurance, government or facility collections. Professionalism, respectful care, and diligent service do not require mandates or policing and are free and easy to deliver to each and every patient.

Patients who choose to invest in their own health have greater expectations. They assume that their physician will provide a service that they cannot obtain on their own. Physicians who act as the authority over patients, rather than an authority of medical information are grossly misled, and their patients suffer the consequences. Patients who choose independent physicians are aware that a physician's duty is to offer advice based on acquired knowledge and experience in a way that involves patient participation. They do not expect to be forced through an "assembly line" of medical processes that may not even include a physician or worse, usually involves a complete stranger who is expected to be "trusted". Invested patients feel responsible for their own health and take that responsibility as a life-long commitment. It is my duty to include patients in the healing process and to lead them in the most effective direction. Most of my recommendations require active participation, rather than passive processes and medications that over time, may have untoward effects. The patients in my practice have goals that they set. The achievement of these goals requires professional medical guidance. I find great relief in not being rushed through a patient visit. My patients understand that the elimination of symptoms is quick and easy, does not always guarantee improved health, and realize that healing takes time and commitment. I enjoy learning about my patients, many of whom have very interesting backgrounds and offer me a learning experience as well. For this, I am grateful. I made the decision to gallantly proceed on my own for the benefit of my patients' well-being and my own and have never looked back.

Again, I am Dr. Lisa Mainier. I am a double board-certified physician. I practice the virtually lost "Art of Medicine" that blends valid, good quality, evidence-based medicine that once gave the physician expert status and authority over information that proved so valuable to his or her patients. As a physician, I am capable of using experience, education, quality scientific evidence and intellect to provide excellent medical care that restores health and improves quality of life. In the practice of medicine, I prefer wisdom, sophistication, and unbiased perception of the problem, coupled with excellent formal education, self-driven investigation, and research rather than the fast-paced, computer-generated, algorithm-based medicine that is prevalent today.

Dr. Lisa's description of medicine and physician care today is reinforced by Dr. Ann Gladstone, DO, in her article "Doctors Are Fleeing the Medical Field. Here's Why." This article was published in The Kevin MD.com, Newsletter, August 10, 2020.

She goes on to say that she can no longer practice the "gold standard" of medical care because at this time it is simply not covered by insurance." There is little time for the practice of medicine--there is only paperwork and red tape."

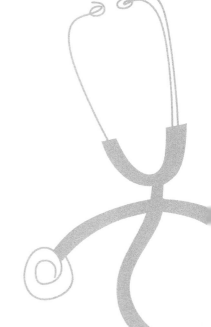

CHAPTER 5

Understanding Medicaid Insurance

As stated before, in 1965 congress passed Title XVIII Medicare and Title XIX Medicaid. Medicaid provides medical coverage based on income levels rather than age requirements. To qualify in the Commonwealth of Pennsylvania, one must be near the poverty level of income. Each state has different eligibility requirements, so if you are living in another state, check that state's requirements.

Pennsylvania Medicaid covers residents who are:

- Aged 19-64 with incomes at or below 133% of the Federal Poverty Level (to put things into context, that equates to about $20,420 for a family of three) or about $12,000 a year for individuals.
- Aged (age 65 and older), blind, or disabled
- In families with children under age 21
- Have special conditions

Nursing Home Care

Previously, we discussed that Medicare pays for skilled services which require care by a registered nurse or physical therapist, occupational therapist or speech therapy daily if they continue to make progress.

Medicare pays in full the first 20 days of skilled care, but for days 21-100, there is a co-pay of $185.50 a day. Unless, an individual can pay privately or has supplemental insurance coverage, they can apply for Medicaid coverage. It must be determined that they are eligible. Once again, they must be living at the poverty level, or about $12,000 a year income. And, In order to be eligible, they must not have any assets. There is a 5-year look-back to determine if someone has given their assets away or spent money excessively (i.e., a trip to Aruba).

The general rule is that if a Senior applies for Medicaid, is deemed otherwise eligible but is found to have gifted assets within the five-year look-back period, then they will be disqualified from receiving benefits for a certain number of months. This is referred to as the Medicaid penalty period.

I have a client that I oversee and manage her care as her family lives out of town. She has been in a nursing home for over 2 months for wound care which is a skilled need, and she has been paying privately for her co-pay since her initial 20 days were completed. Ultimately, she will have paid $200,000. And then she will be eligible for Medicaid.

Once someone no longer can benefit from skilled care and continues to need nursing home care, they must pay privately and spend down or apply for Medicaid to stay in that nursing home.

Often, families will seek an attorney who specializes in elder law to protect their assets and not have to spend down all their funds. This is a very personal decision. My wife decided that when her mother needed nursing home care, her mother's money would pay for her care and spend down prior to going on Medicaid.

I would suggest that you consult an elder law attorney to provide information and to determine any alternative strategies to protect your assets.

Alternatives to Nursing Home Care Act 150.

If you have a physical disability, the Pennsylvania state-funded Act 150 program may be an alternative solution. If eligible, an individual can continue to live at home with support and services being provided. This is funded through the Pa. Department of Human Services and should be consulted regarding the application process.

Qualified individuals receive:

- Personal Assistance Services (aid and attendant care)
- Personal Emergency Response System
- Service Coordination

Act 150 eligibility is based on a level of care assessment, a financial eligibility determination and program eligibility. Financial eligibility is determined through Medicaid eligibility, which is, again, having an income at poverty level with the five-year look back.

Home and Community Based Services

If you are 60 and over you can be eligible for Home and Community Based Services which are similar services to the above by once again qualifying for Medicaid.

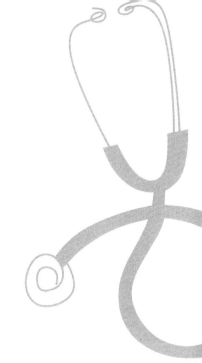

CHAPTER 6

Obama Care or the Affordable Care Act

What is Obamacare?

The Patient Protection and Affordable Care Act (ACA)– commonly referred to as the Affordable Care Act and also known as Obamacare – is a sweeping piece of legislation passed by the 111th Congress and signed into law by President Barack Obama in 2010. The law was intended to improve the affordability and quality of health insurance in the United States

Prior to this bill being signed there were 36 million people in the US that had no insurance or were under insured. These individuals and family members earned an income that was above the qualifying threshold to apply for Medicaid and yet they worked in places or owned a small business that did not pay for their health insurance. According to www.Healthinsurance.org, 50 million people are better off because of the ACA.

Some of the most significant statistics about the Affordable Care Act are:

- More than 9 million Americans who are receiving premium subsidies in the exchanges find their coverage affordable. The average full-price premium is $594/month in 2019, but the average subsidy amount ($514/month) covers most of the average premium.
- People who are (or want to be) self-employed wouldn't have been able to qualify for and/ or afford a privately purchased health insurance plan without the ACA's guaranteed-issue provisions and premium subsidies.

- People with pre-existing conditions gained access to an employer-sponsored plan after being uninsured for 63+ days. HIPAA guaranteed that they could enroll in the employer-sponsored plan, but there were waiting periods for pre-existing conditions. The ACA eliminated those waiting periods.

- In addition, many people could not get coverage because they had a pre-existing condition. This act allows these individuals to obtain coverage. This provided much needed healthcare assistance to many people.

- People who exhausted their medical benefits due to a serious chronic condition were now eligible to continue to have medical benefits.

- According to the Congressional Budget Office, the 2020 budget in the United States, 6.6 trillion dollars were being spent and the revenue was 3.2 trillion dollars. This is called deficit spending! Medicare was 3.7% of the GDP or 769 billion dollars and Medicaid was 2.2% of the GDP or 458 billion dollars. This compares to defense spending of 778 billion dollars.

Medicare, Medicaid, Social Security and Defense comprise the largest amounts of money spent annually. Obama Care has been controversial because it has increased additional costs to the health care budget. Until this country decides that access to health care is an entitlement for all Americans, the healthcare budget will continue to be controversial.

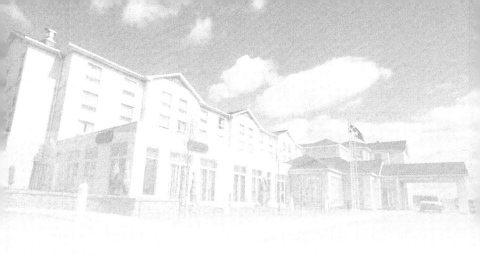

CHAPTER 7

Nursing Homes

In a previous chapter, I discussed how nursing homes originally started as religious based homes providing quality care for the poor. They now have evolved into largely profit oriented poor-quality facilities. Approximately, only 10-20% of the facilities across the country are of excellent quality. As a nursing home administrator for over 25 years, it saddens me to say that I have seen the quality of care provided by this industry deteriorate. Most administrators hide behind the excuse that the facilities do not receive enough reimbursement from the insurance and governmental agencies. However, this does not excuse them from their poor quality of patient care.

The JAA, (where I was employed and where I helped design the nursing home programs) closed its nursing home using the excuse that the reimbursement was inadequate! Yet the other religious based facilities are thriving and providing quality care with the same reimbursement.

Nursing homes across the country are inspected annually by their State Department of Health and licensed for Medicare and Medicaid reimbursement. Because they are licensed for both they must comply with federal guidelines as well as the state. The federal guidelines are developed and overseen by CMS (Center for Medicare and Medicaid Services). If they have a poor inspection, or there are founded complaints, they are inspected more often, until their deficiencies have been resolved.

Every resident or family member has the right to complain about care to the Area on Aging Ombudsman Program and/or the Department of Health. Often, they are afraid to complain, for fear of retaliation. I encourage everyone to complain if they cannot get their conflict resolved at the facility. Complaints are confidential and when the Department of Health visits unannounced they usually look at similar cases along with the complainant.

As an administrator, I would always make rounds daily, keep my door open, have a suggestion box and attend resident council (a monthly meeting which was attended by the residents and or families). It was much easier to resolve a complaint at the facility level than at the Department of Health investigating level.

I also started a welcome program to the facility, where I or one of the department heads would greet the resident on admission and visit them daily for the first week to 10 days to answer their questions or complaints. This way the resident knew they had someone who acted as their internal advocate from the beginning of their stay.

I would suggest that if the facility you are considering or are currently residing in does not follow these practices, then you probably should be considering a different facility.

You can learn how any nursing home in the country is rated by vising https://www.cms.gov/ and reviewing nursing home comparisons. Nursing homes are currently rated on several areas: the results of their inspections, complaints, quality measures and staffing. This rating is on a 5-star system with 5 stars being the best and 1 star the worst.

Substandard Quality of Care

Substandard Quality of Care is a technical regulatory term which means that one or more requirements under the federal regulations 42CFR 483.13 (resident behavior and facility practices), 42CFR 483.15 (quality of life), or 42CFR 483.25 (quality of care) were not met. The substandard quality of care ranges from a degree constituting immediate jeopardy to resident health or safety, and a scope of pattern or widespread actual harm, or a widespread potential for more than minimal harm. A finding of substandard quality of care indicates that the nursing home was found to have had a significant deficiency (or deficiencies), which the home must correct quickly to protect the health and safety of residents. The government specifies a maximum time frame for correction of the deficiencies. That could be anywhere from immediately to several weeks depending on the scope and severity of the deficiency.

According to the Kaiser Foundation, more than one-third of nursing homes certified by Medicare or Medicaid have relatively low overall star ratings of 1 or 2 stars, accounting for 39 percent of all nursing home residents. Conversely, 45 percent of nursing homes have overall ratings of 4 or 5 stars, accounting for 41 percent of all nursing home residents.

For-profit nursing homes, which are more prevalent, tend to have lower star ratings than non-profit nursing homes, because for profit facilities usually have lower staffing levels.

In 11 states, at least 40 percent of nursing homes have relatively low ratings (1 or 2 stars). In 22 states and the District of Columbia, at least 50 percent of the nursing homes in the state have relatively high overall ratings (4 or 5 stars). States that have higher proportions of low-income seniors tend to have lower-rated nursing homes.

Nursing home deficiencies are broken down into:

- immediate jeopardy to resident health or safety
- actual harm that is not immediate jeopardy
- no actual harm with potential for more than minimal harm but not immediate jeopardy
- no actual harm with potential for minimal harm

HOLD THE PRESSES!

Just as I was going to send this to my editor, *McKnight Long Term Care News* April 6, 2022 published an article, by Danielle Brown

BREAKING: US NURSING HOME SYSTEM, "INEFFECTIVE" "UNSUSTAINABLE"

National Academies Report says "The way in which the United States finances, delivers, and regulates care in a nursing home setting is inefficient, fragmented and unsustainable.

The report's goal is to make high quality person centered and equitable care a "reality " for the nursing home residents.

Once again, It's time to blow it all up because the system is broken!

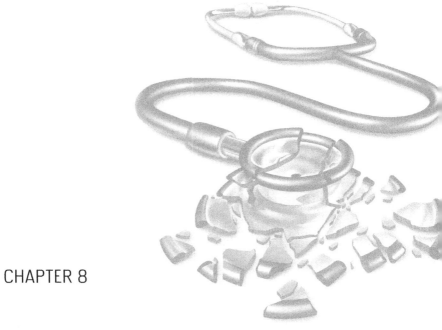

CHAPTER 8

Nursing Home Abuse and Neglect

Nursing Home Abuse:

Nursing home abuse occurs when caretakers harm residents at long-term care facilities or at home. Both intentional and unintentional harm may be considered abuse. It can result in patient trauma, medical emergencies, and even death.

Sadly, nursing home abuse is a prevalent problem due to issues such as understaffing, improper training, and employee burnout. These factors can cause staff members to focus their anger on the people they should care for or offer a delayed response to urgent situations such as patient falls or strokes.

Fortunately, there are steps that you can take if an elder person you love has suffered from nursing home abuse. First, you can keep them safe by reporting abuse to proper authorities like the police, Adult Protective Services, the Department of Health and an attorney.

These Statistics are frightening, according to Nursing Home Abuse Justice:

- As many as 1 in 3 older people have been victims of nursing home abuse. Further, 2 in 3 staff members surveyed by the World Health Organization (WHO) claimed they had abused or neglected residents.

- A study from 2012 found that as many as 85% of assisted living facilities reported at least one case of abuse or neglect — but this number may actually be much higher.

- In a 2019 NPR report, the Office of Inspector General (OIG) found that 97% of nursing home abuse cases across 5 states were not reported to local law enforcement as required.

Types of Abuse in Nursing Homes

The term "nursing home abuse" often seems to imply physical injuries. However, it may also include sexual battery and emotional harm and all of the other issues noted below. It's important to know which type of nursing home abuse your loved one is suffering from so you can properly help them.

Physical Abuse: If nursing home staff members knowingly cause physical harm to residents, they are committing abuse. Common examples of physical abuse include pushing, kicking, and hitting.

Emotional Abuse: Emotional abuse includes any type of action that harms an older person's psychological well-being. Examples of emotional abuse include staff yelling at residents or taunting them. Staff members may also try to isolate the resident from friends and family. While these actions may not leave physical marks, they can be just as harmful. Nursing home residents that suffer from emotional abuse may experience anxiety and depression.

Sexual Abuse: Those who live in nursing homes can suffer from sexual battery. This type of abuse includes any form of unwanted sexual activity. A 2017 CNN report explored cases where nursing home residents had been sexually abused by staff members. In total, the report found over 1,000 nursing home facilities across the country received citations for mismanaging sexual abuse cases.

Financial Exploitation: This includes theft of personal possessions and/or family members or friends spending their money without their permission.

Nursing Home Neglect: Some nursing home residents may be left unattended for extended periods of time and put in danger. Nursing home neglect can lead to malnutrition, infections, and bedsores, among other problems.

Also, nursing home residents are at risk of staff mismanaging their money, putting them at risk of elder financial abuse. For example, the Chicago Sun-Times reported that two nursing home employees stole over $750,000 from a resident with dementia before they were caught.

The National Center for Victims of Crime breakdown of nursing home abuse complaints is as follows:

- 27.4% – Physical abuse
- 22.1% – Resident-on-resident abuse (physical or sexual)
- 19.4% – Psychological abuse
- 15.3% – Gross neglect
- 7.9% – Sexual abuse
- 7.9% – Financial exploitation

Nursing home abuse is one part of the larger problem with elder abuse. As many as 5,000,000 people are affected by elder abuse every single year, according to the National Center of Abuse

Like all other crimes, not every case of nursing home abuse gets reported, and researchers are trying to determine exact figures. This is further complicated by the fact that some seniors may be unwilling — or unable — to report their experiences.

As a Nationally Certified Patient Advocate, I have known of clients who have been abused in nursing homes and at home. Several clients have developed pressure sores because staff have not been attentive. If someone is bedridden, they are to be turned and re-positioned every 2 hours. Special cushioning should be used as well as a specialty bed with an air mattress providing alternating pressure. It is most important to visit your loved one every day and get to know the staff, thus developing a positive relationship with them. Also, the staff becomes aware that someone is monitoring the patient's care. If you cannot provide this, then one should consider hiring a patient advocate to monitor your loved one's care. I am a licensed nursing home administrator and with my credentials comes improved quality care for your loved one since I will be monitoring the care. I try to partner with the facility to improve the care for my clients. If the facilities do not want to cooperate, I don't mind confrontation.

I had a client hire me because the patient's daughter felt her father was not getting the care or attention that was required. They would get him dressed in the morning and put him in a wheelchair and place him in front of the nurses' station all day because he was determined to be a fall risk. No one would interact with him during the day except for saying hello as they passed by.

This is a common practice: any resident identified as a fall risk is seated in front of the nurse's station all day so that the nurses can keep an "eye" on them! Typically, there is no interaction with the residents, and you see them slumped over in their wheelchair usually sleeping because of boredom! I consider this neglect of care although usually no one gets called out for it. If you should see this behavior when you are visiting a nursing home to determine if your loved one should go there, turn around and walk out. Going back to my client, not only was he not getting care at the nurses' station, but he was also not getting any restorative care.

Restorative care is provided by nursing when the resident no longer qualifies for therapy. It is needed so that the resident does not decline. Restorative care includes having a nurse walk with the resident. If the resident is bed ridden, nursing provides active and passive range of motion for the resident's limbs. Not only does this benefit the resident but it benefits the facility because they get reimbursed at a higher rate for providing this care.

However, this facility was not providing this care, although they claimed they were because the resident was eating by moving his hand and arm to feed himself. I told the director of nursing that was not the definition of restorative care according to the government regulations and if they were calling what they were doing restorative, they were committing fraud! When the daughter transferred her father out of the facility, I reported them to the Department of Health for poor care and fraud.

In one facility, I was brought in for training because on their past survey, residents told the surveyors that they were being yelled at by staff. The facility was given a deficiency for potential widespread verbal abuse and potential harm. Since these episodes were unwitnessed but reported, the deficiency was for potential, not actual harm. They were required to have mandatory abuse in-service training which I provided to every employee. During the training, I discovered that some of the employees felt exactly like the residents. They were bullied by other employees.

This resulted in trying to change a culture by building teamwork and respect.

A Patient Advocate Colleague's Personal Experience

Becoming A Patient Advocate by **Anne Llewellyn, MS, BHSA, RN, CCM, CRRN, CMGT-BC, FCM**

As a nurse of over 40 years, I always thought I was a patient advocate. I would be the one who stood up for my patients when I worked in an inner-city emergency department in Philadelphia or stayed late to talk to a family member of a patient who almost died in our intensive care unit. I was the one who gave the homeless patient a sandwich, a cup of coffee, and a blanket and let him sleep t in the emergency department waiting room on a cold winter night. I thought this was what being an advocate was – and it is, but there is more to it.

My Story

On a bright sunny day in November of 2014, I was driving home from an eye doctor's appointment when I made a turn and hit the curb. The tire blew out, so I had to call my husband to pick me up. He did, and when he arrived, he asked me if I was ok. I said I felt fine. He said that I did not look right and thought we should go to the emergency department – so off we went.

I was seen by the emergency room doctor, who ordered a CAT Scan. I had the test, and when the doctor came in and closed the door, I knew the news was not good. He explained that the CAT Scan showed that I had a brain tumor. He suggested that I be admitted, and they would have a neurosurgeon see me the next day to decide what to do. At that moment – I knew my life would change forever.

I called a few friends – a nurse case manager and a patient advocate colleague and told them what happened. They said they would come over to the hospital the next day. The neurosurgeon came by, and when he saw my friends in the room, he said, 'who are they? Attorneys?' My husband said no; they were nurses who worked with my wife. He said, 'ok, they can stay, but they can't take any notes.' I thought this was very strange but tried to listen to what he was there to tell me. He went on to tell us what he saw on the CAT Scan and what he wanted to do. He said he would take me to the OR, drill a hole into my head, take out a piece of the tumor, analyze it, and then connect me to an oncologist. Any questions?

I said, "Doctor, who would you have to do this procedure if it was your wife or daughter? "He told me: 'I'm the best.' Without looking at me, he said, 'Ok, we will get you set up for the OR tomorrow' and walked out the door.

After the doctor left, my friends talked to my husband and said they would like to see if they could do some research as they did not think I was in the most appropriate hospital to have brain surgery. I was in a small community hospital closest to my home. My husband told them to see what they could do. They called him later in the day and told him they had gotten a neurosurgeon at the University of Miami who agreed to take the case. My husband asked my nurse to see the neurosurgeon. The nurse brought him on the phone. My husband told the doctor we would go to the University of Miami for treatment and would he discharge me. My husband gave him the doctor's name, so they knew I had a doctor to see once I left. The doctor was very upset and said that it was not necessary to go to another hospital, that he could do the surgery. My husband explained we did not think we were in the right place and preferred to go to the University of Miami. He discharged me and left the room shaking his head.

After I was discharged, I went down to the University of Miami and met with the 2nd neurosurgeon, who told me what he would do. It was like what the 1st Neurosurgeon told me he would do, but with more confidence and compassion for me as the patient. I felt he had a much better bedside manner, and I instantly trusted him. I felt safer with him.

He did the procedure, and once the biopsy results were back, the neurosurgeon referred me to a hematologist who specialized in the type of tumor I had. I saw the hematologist/oncologist and was told that I had a large central nervous system lymphoma that was not operable. He said I would need chemotherapy to shrink the tumor. If chemo did not work, he said he would have to add radiation, but the protocol he was putting me on showed great success with this type of tumor. He said I would need to go into the hospital every two weeks for chemo as the protocol was a combination of several powerful chemotherapy agents, and I needed to be monitored. On New Year's Eve, I was admitted to the hospital and stayed for four days.

After the 3rd round of chemo, the doctor wanted me to get an MRI. I was nervous as a result would dictate my course of treatment. The doctor came to my room and told us the tumor was GONE! My husband and I did not understand this but were cautiously relieved. The doctor said the protocol he had me on is meant to work quickly if it would work at all. He told me I still had to finish another

12 rounds, but at this point, it looked like I was out of the woods.

As I recovered and began to understand what had happened to me, I realized I was fortunate to get out of the first hospital and go to the University of Miami. I knew this would not have happened if it were not for my two friends, who recognized I was not in the right setting and advocated for me to get to an academic medical center to see a team that was up to date on the latest protocols and treatments for the tumor I had. I realized what a patient advocate could do for a person who was thrust into the complex healthcare system.

The doctor at the first hospital was right, he could do brain surgery, and he would send me to an oncologist. But would they have put me on the protocol that I was put on by the hematologist who saw me at Sylvester Comprehensive Cancer Center? I will never know – they would do what they could – but would it work? No one at the first hospital would tell me to go somewhere else as they could treat me. Since this day, I have said that the healthcare system is built for the healthcare system, not the people who use it.

As I recovered and had more visits to the Sylvester Comprehensive Cancer Center, I saw so many people who came to the clinic alone, who did not have anyone with them. My husband and I often wondered how they did this alone? It was at this point that I knew I wanted to do more. I wanted to help people thrust into the healthcare system realize they needed to have someone with them to be their advocate. My role is to help people have a voice, ask questions, and make sure their treatment aligns with their goals. I wanted people to know they could ask for a 2nd opinion and not be worried that the doctor would be upset. I wanted to help people learn how to advocate for themselves and be an active member of THEIR health care team.

Before getting sick, I knew what patient advocates were. This experience helped me understand what a patient advocate was from a personal standpoint. My experience made it real – that everyone needs an advocate when they enter the healthcare system. The system is designed for the healthcare system and not the people who use it. Having advocates as I did with my two friends and husband helped me get to the academic center that saved my life.

Once we were in active treatment, my husband was my advocate. He had no training as an advocate but learned how to do this by talking to my two friends. They told him to get a binder and keep track of what the doctors said. They encouraged him to listen, ask questions if he did not understand something, and make sure that we were comfortable with the treatment and care.

My husband put what they said into practice. It was amazing how many times the notes he took came in handy. A few times, a new resident or a new Fellow would come into my room when I was in the hospital and say they wanted to try something. My husband would ask, did you check with Dr. Lossos as he did not mention any changes. They would leave, make a call, and come back and say they would not be making any changes as it was not part of the protocol. If my husband was not there and did not speak up, who knows what could have happened. He asked a nurse what medication she was giving me a few times. If he did not recognize the name, he would ask her to check to make sure she was giving me the correct medication. Often, the nurse would come back and tell him he was right – that medication was for another patient. Having my husband by my side kept me safe.

As I started to think about going back to work, I knew I had to use my clinical skills and experience as a cancer patient to educate people about who advocates were, why they were necessary, and how to find one. I also took on a few cases myself as a nurse advocate. Being a nurse advocate kept me grounded and allowed me to see how my work could help others by being part of their care.

Over the years, I have learned that being an advocate is hard work because most people don't know who advocates are or how they help the patient and the family. People don't understand why they need to pay for an advocate when they have a doctor and an entire health care team to help them. To explain this, I decided to write a blog to use my examples and experience to show people what an advocate is and why they are so crucial through storytelling.

I started to put together programs to teach people (patients and their families) how they could be advocates for each other and find one if they wound their cases were too complex for them to handle. My writings are also designed to educate the health care team so they would know who advocates are and the value they bring to all stakeholders.

Why trying to explain why an advocate is so important, I often ask: would you go into a court of law without an attorney? So why would you go into the healthcare system without an advocate with you to help you understand how the system works? An advocate ensures you have a voice and the courage to ask questions that are important to you. An advocate gives you another set of ears as it allows someone to hear what the doctor, nurses, or therapist say to you when they explain your plan of care. Having an advocate reminds you of what was said after the appointment. They will remind you that you want to ask a question or talk about another care plan like the one that is not working for you.

Advocates can be family members, trusted friends, or paid professionals. They are someone who cares for you and looks out for you in a complex and fragmented system.

I love what I am doing, and I love that it helps others understand who advocates are and why they have an essential role in our healthcare system for the patient, the family, and all health care team members.

To learn more about patient advocacy, here is an article that looks at the history and trends in patient advocacy; History and Trends in Patient Advocate: an interesting article from a leader in patient advocacy https://aphadvocates.org/assets/History-Trends-CSA-Schuler-12.21.pdf.

If you are a patient or family member looking to find an advocate, visit Greater National Advocate at https://www.gnanow.org. If you want to become a patient advocate, there are training programs you can investigate. A few companies provide education to those who wish to become patient/health advocates.

- **The Bridge Health Advocacy Program:** https://bridgehealthadvocates.com/bha-advocacy-academy
- **Care Excellence: https://www.careexcellenceinstitute.com**
- **Practice Up** https://practiceuponline.com
- **Assumption College Health Advocacy Program** https://www.assumption.edu/graduate/health-advocacy
- **Pulse Center for Patient Advocacy**: https://pulsecenterforpatientsafety.org
- **Campaign Zero:** https://campaignzero.org
- **National Association of Health Care Advocacy: They are a professional organization with a new mentoring program. You must be a member, but membership will open many doors. To learn more,**

visit the NAHAC website at https://www. nahac.com/nahac-mentoring-program.

- **Nurse Advocate Entrepreneur** http://www. nurseadvocateentrepreneur.com

Through Ann's narrative what was apparent is that Ann had the right to get a second opinion and choose the course of treatment which was best for her. She became a patient advocate to assist others in knowing their rights and helping them to get second opinions if necessary and help then know alternative courses of treatment so they can make intelligent decisions about their care.

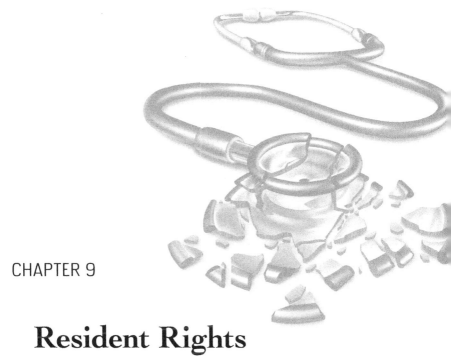

CHAPTER 9

Resident Rights and Restraints

Residents have the right to be free of restraints. Restraints can be considered physical and/or chemical and are defined as restricting movement. Reference: *Journal of Medical Ethics* "Use of Physical Restraints in Nursing Homes—A clinical and ethical consideration."

Physical risks.

Over the last few years, a consensus has been building about the physical risks associated with the application of physical restraint to older people, the physical consequences of which are:

- bruises
- decubitus ulcers
- respiratory complications
- urinary incontinence and constipation
- undernutrition
- impaired muscle strength and balance
- increased agitation
- decreased cardiovascular endurance
- increased risk for mortality

Side Rails in beds are also considered restraints. One might think that siderails prevent falls. However, this is not the case. Instead, side rails cause injuries and possible death.

According to the National Library of Medicine:

Deaths described are categorized into three types: (1) 70% were entrapments between the mattress and a rail so that the face was pressed against the mattress, (2) 18% were entrapment and compression of the neck within the rails, and (3) 12% were deaths caused by being trapped by the rails after sliding partially off the bed and having the neck flexed or the chest compressed.

In September of 2017, a resident was asphyxiated from an incident in which his neck was trapped in bed rails, in a prominent nursing facility in Pittsburgh, Pa. The facility was cited for causing actual harm and was severely penalized by the Pa. Department of Health.

Chemical Restraints

Chemical Restraints are the use of psychotropic medication to sedate residents and inhibit them from acting out. Some of these include:

Typical antipsychotics
- chlorpromazine (Thorazine);
- fluphenazine (Prolixin);

- haloperidol (Haldol);
- perphenazine (Trilafon);
- thioridazine (Mellaril)

Typical anti-anxiety

- alprazolam (Xanax);
- clonazepam (Klonopin);
- diazepam (Valium)
- lorazepam (Ativan)

If your loved one is on an antipsychotic and does not have a diagnosis that warrants its use, then you should know if it is being used as a chemical restraint or being used to sedate your loved one for staff convenience.

The common anti-anxiety medications above also cannot be given without a corresponding diagnosis.

For the facility to use a chemical restraint there must be a physician's order. In addition, you must be told the side effects and given permission for usage.

In a New York Times article written September 12, 2021, titled "False Diagnoses Hide Drugging of Nursing Home Patients," a federal oversight agency said that nearly one third of the residents with the diagnosis of schizophrenia who were given psychoactive drugs had no medical record of being treated for such condition. The side effects of these drugs include:

- Increased dependence and functional decline
- Loss of memory
- Agitation
- Withdrawal and depression
- Loss of mobility and strength
- Increased risk of accidents and falls
- Low blood pressure
- Muscle disorders
- Adverse drug effects

Along with these side effects. The Nursing Home Abuse Guide stated 15 million deaths a year occur in nursing homes and 88% of residents who have dementia are prescribed an anti-psychotic drug.

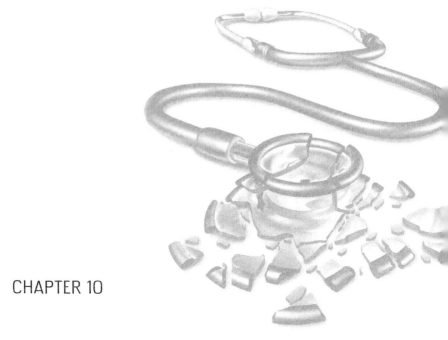

CHAPTER 10

Nursing Home Fraud

In the September 21, 2021, edition of *McKnight's Long Term Care News*, the headline read: "Approved: Consulate Health Care to pay just $4.5 million of $258 million judgment in inherited upcoding case."

The settlement was the result of a judgement rendered in a therapy upcoding case. Six of the Consulate Health Care facilities in Florida filed bankruptcy, stating they couldn't pay the 258-million-dollar judgement. Therapy upcoding simply means that the facility that was recording therapy minutes did not occur to get a higher level of reimbursement. This was commonplace for facilities as well as therapy companies.

Channel 4 Action News in Pittsburgh, on February 25, 2021, reported that a nursing home manager was indicted in Mt. Lebanon for falsifying records to make it appear that the facility met federal and state staffing requirements. This investigation came after the FBI served search warrants for 6 months. The conspiracy deprived residents of patient care by inflating nursing hours, falsifying nursing hours, and other schemes. This went on for approximately 2 years from 2018 to 2020. These facilities were owned by the same group, Comprehensive Healthcare.

Unbeknownst to me, I unfortunately served as an interim administrator in one of the facilities owned by Comprehensive Healthcare for about 4 months and I called their operation the PONZI SCHEME.

There was not enough staff, supplies or equipment to take care of the residents. The owners would not allow the facility to deny an admission unless they approved it. There is a saying in this industry called "Putting Heads In Beds".

Their bottom line was keeping the census as high as possible. They took obese clients which required special beds and equipment and more staff for lifting as well as clients who were drug and alcohol addicted. The staff was ill-prepared and untrained to take care of them! Many dedicated staff left because they were tired of working short-handed or not having the equipment they needed. When equipment was ordered it was denied by their purchasing department.

It is a regulation that every room has a clock in it so the resident can maintain their reality by knowing the time and date. There were no clocks in any room when I arrived. I ordered clocks and purchasing denied the request. When I sent the order back stating that this was a federal regulation for each room to have a wall clock in the room, it was denied again. These clocks cost about $20. The overall purchase would have cost the facility about $500. Before I left the facility as its interim administrator, the medical director fell out of a chair at the nurse's station. Fortunately, he did not get hurt. The mechanism that raises and lowers the chair was broken so that when he sat in it, the chair did not stay in the position. It automatically lowered, and he fell. I ordered another chair; it was denied, at which point I demanded the director of purchasing who was a cousin to the owners to come sit in the chair. When she refused, I got her to order the chair and I won $20 from the medical director as he bet me that I could not get another chair!

On May 8, 2020, the Pittsburgh Post Gazette published a column stating that State Representative Conor Lamb, D-Mt. Lebanon, demanded a federal investigation of the Brighton Rehabilitation and Wellness Center in Beaver County, another facility owned and run by Comprehensive Healthcare. "This is a sign of growing impatience with how Pennsylvania health officials have handled the state's worst nursing home outbreak of COVID-19, which has claimed 71 lives."

Mr. Lamb, in an interview, said he felt compelled to ask federal officials to intervene after he was notified last weekend that the facility's managers were cited for failing to wash their hands and to properly clean equipment that comes into contact with residents who have been infected with COVID 19 and those who had not. Finally, around the same time period, the Attorney General of Pennsylvania was opening a criminal probe of Brighton Nursing Center in Beaver County as well as other facilities.

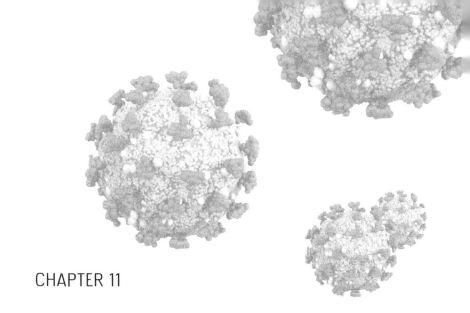

CHAPTER 11

COVID 19: Three Years of Hell and Counting

On March 13, 2020, (Friday the 13th), all of the nursing homes in Pa. were notified that they were no longer permitted to allow visitation. In addition, nursing home residents were relegated to their rooms and were no longer allowed to congregate for meals or activities . The President of the United States was providing very little direction or resources to the country or to health care facilities. In fact, he kept saying the Pandemic will be over soon. This left the states to rely on their resources to deal with Covid 19.

To make matters worse, the former Governor of New York, Cuomo, mandated that nursing homes take back Covid 19 patients so the hospitals could handle the overflow. He then hid the data about deaths of nursing home residents for many months.

In a McKnight Publication, October 21, 2021, John O'Connor, vice president of McKnight Long Term Care News, wrote a blog entitled: "Do Seniors Even Count?" In this blog Mr. O'Conner revealed that the new governor who replaced Mario Cuomo, Kathy Hochul, reported that Mario Cuomo under- reported nursing home deaths by nearly 12,000 deaths. He was never held accountable for his dereliction of duty. Instead, he stepped down because the New York attorney general, Letitia James, alleged that Cuomo sexually harassed 11 women causing a "hostile work environment," a year after he had under-reported the nursing home deaths. Mr. O'Connor concludes "that there is something disturbing about the relative value that's placed on Seniors".

In a March 25, 2020 NPR report on the Coronavirus, there was concern about distribution of COVID 19 supplies to the public and health care facilities. The story was titled: "Trump Resists Using Wartime Law (The Defense Act) to Get and Distribute Coronavirus Supplies." Many governors and health officials had been pleading with President Trump to use his authority under the Defense Production Act to get the federal government more directly involved in the buying and distribution of items like ventilators and face masks — items that have been in short supply, with states competing for them.

While Trump had designated ventilators and protective equipment as essential under the law, he did not use the act to force companies to produce certain items.

As a result, hospitals and nursing homes were forced to use garbage bags as Personal Protective Equipment, face masks that had very little protection and infected staff continuing to work because there were not any procedures or equipment to screen them. During that period there were 131,000 who died with Covid 19 according to federal data, making up nearly a quarter of the US deaths due to Covid. Talk about the question, "Do Seniors Count?"

One of my clients discusses his personal journey dealing with his 93-year-old impaired mother during Covid.

—⊩—o❀o—⊩—

When I arrived in Pittsburgh after my 93-year-old mother fell in her home and broke her leg, I had little idea of what I would be responsible for during the next fourteen months. The COVID pandemic was spiking. The day after her surgery I was told by the surgical team representative I had twenty-four hours to remove her from the hospital. I was shocked and confused, and really did not know what to do. I was told I had two choices: take her to a "facility," or take her home. At that time rehab facilities were centers for the COVID outbreak. Visitations were not allowed. Therefore the choice was easy, though seemingly impossible. I needed to take her home to the house where she had lived for sixty-five years. I would have to turn that home into a facility for post-operative care and rehab.

Caregiving, I was to find out, is not an easy job. What's more, the caregiver business that had sent two live-in caregivers for many years alerted me they were short on staff. Their representative, in fact, counseled that I should take my mother to a facility.

Luckily a doctor friend in town recommended several part time caregivers and nurses she had vetted for her parents. I was tasked with putting together a team. The surgery was successful. For some reason, however, after several months, her condition worsened. My mother had pain in her abdomen. It worsened when she urinated. After many trips back to the hospital she was diagnosed with bladder cancer. She died just after her 95th birthday.

Post-op she lived the entire time in her house, in her first-floor den, in a rented hospital bed. She was able, with help, to amble to the kitchen for meals, until the caregivers told me they would need to use a wheelchair. There came a point she could no longer feed herself. The entire time caregivers had to wash and dress her.

Through it all the institutional medical community was of little to no help in her care. There are many stories including not being able to receive intravenous hydration in the home as she was diagnosed as chronically dehydrated.

I met Jeff Weinberg of Caregiver Champion as I was looking for a manager for the caregivers at home. I was exhausted and needed to take a break. At the same time I was told we should begin Hospice care. Every conversation with Jeff Weinberg, the director of Caregiver Champion, as well as all the professional referrals he made, including the hospice care group we ultimately accepted, were extremely helpful to the family and beneficial to my mother.

With so many issues arising concerning different courses of action to take, it was amazing to the family how little help—both for my mother, the care givers, and the family at large—was received from cancer specialists, gerontologists, and gynecological professionals in the hospital system. At the same time it was amazing to find help for both physical and emotional issues as they arose through Caregiver Champion. The professionals I met through Caregiver Champion took the time to listen and to respond at our time of need.

The Jewish philosopher Martin Buber wrote in his famous book "I and Thou" that there exist two types of human relationships. One is where we treat the other as an object. He named these "I-It" relationships. The second type is when we treat the other as a special creation as ourselves—"I-Thou." In the "I-Thou" relationship we are able to include both the objective and the personal. End of life moments for elderly parents include medical, emotional, and spiritual realities. The human resources Caregiver Champion provided, at a very difficult time in the life my family, even at a time of a pandemic, stood out from all others in that they included both I-Thou and I-It experiences. This should be true for any care giving "facility."

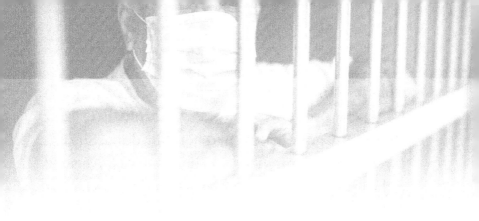

CHAPTER 12

Social Isolation or as I call it: "The Second Pandemic"

Not only were there actual deaths due to Covid 19, but there were also many deaths of nursing home patients due to social isolation and a medical condition known as Failure to Thrive.

On March 13, 2020, my wife Dee was told she could no longer visit her mother, Sarah, in a nursing home. My wife had visited her mother every day for 2 years. After only 3-4 months, my mother-in-law Sarah passed away due to her social isolation and condition, Failure to Thrive. Sarah was a very proud woman, at 97 years old. Every day she got up, got dressed, had her hair done. She enjoyed a weekly manicure. When she was relegated to her room and could no longer see my wife, nor her friends in the facility at mealtime, she began to give up. She could not recognize the gowned and masked staff caring for her. She refused to eat and no longer cared about her appearance.

One might think that Sarah was in poor health, but that was not the case. She was alert and oriented and her physical health was good. She had a constant Blood Pressure of 110/80. I used to say she didn't have high blood pressure, she caused it! The reason she lived in a nursing home was due to her unsteady balance and gait. She had fallen several times causing very serious injuries. We kept her home with 24-hour care until her available money was depleted. After a year we spent well over $100,000. The only way she could get 24-hour care was through Medicaid in a nursing home.

The facility we chose had an exceptional staff but the administrator was non-caring about staff, residents, and visiting family members. This administrator rarely left her office. When the Covid virus hit, she did not communicate the conditions to family members. Initially, the only way to find out about your loved one was to try to call the nursing home and talk with a staff member.

About a month after the facility required no in-person visitation, nursing homes began permitting window or door visitation. However, this administrator would not permit it and offered no explanation. In fact, she would not answer her telephone and would tell the receptionist she is unavailable. This exacerbated the social isolation. The night my mother-in-law was dying a very kind male nurse called to tell my wife that Sarah was dying. Dee told the nurse that she was coming in to see her. The nurse then called the administrator who denied visitation.

Dee than called the medical director who attempted to call the administrator. Again, this administrator refused to answer her phone, so the medical director told Dee to come in. When she arrived, she put on gloves, a protective gown, and mask to see her mother. The nurse who had called said he was reading the Bible to Sarah before Dee arrived. What a wonderful compassionate thing to do! Dee was permitted about 10 minutes with her dying mother when a nurse knocked on the door and told her the administrator required her to leave. Several hours later, her mother passed away, alone.

However, the story does not stop there. About a week later Dee received an email from the assistant administrator, not stating any sympathy but asking when she was going to pick up her mother's belongings. And if they were not picked up, they would be donated! How cold and cruel can someone get?

So far, I have spoken about lies, fraud and abuse. In my opinion, an administrator who cannot demonstrate compassion and caring and just considers the residents "Heads in beds", is just as criminal as fraud and abuse! Social Isolation is a silent killer.

In a Washington Post article titled "A daughter's choice: Her Mom Didn't Have Covid 19. But Isolation Seemed to Be Killing Her," Geriatrician Michael Wasserman said cases of neglect, have gone unnoticed because when visitors were barred, residents lost their most important watchdogs, their families. At the same time, the mass shutdown created a deep social isolation that experts say has contributed to soaring rates of depression and anxiety and a general loss of the will to live. As a health care patient advocate, I tried to raise awareness of this second pandemic.

My congressman, whose father died in a terrible nursing home incident, arranged for a meeting with me and several state officials from the Department of Health to review the impact of social isolation. They empathized with me, but their concern was that nursing homes follow the state and federal regulations. The regulations were only concerned with the residents' physical wellbeing, such as infection control and bed sores. There was no regulation dealing with social isolation, except abuse. However, if I pressed my case regarding Dee's mother, the whole nursing home network would have to be charged and the Department of Health was not going to investigate every facility in the state.

In meeting with them, my whole presentation was focused on not only the physical aspects of care but the psychosocial aspects of care as well. I was then contacted by a local health care foundation who said they were working on a similar scenario, and they would put me on their research committee. However, there was no follow up. I was contacted by Christine Sorenson, KDKA news anchor, who was appalled to hear what was going on. She described it as living in a prison and I added that health care was probably much better there! To view this entire KDKA-TV interview visit my website, www.caregiverchampionadvocate.com.

I have cited a lack of care and caring for the most part in hospitals and nursing homes, and in the end, driving profits determine the basis of care. These changes in health care and caring have led me to become a health care patient advocate. As a health care advocate, I tried to raise awareness of this second pandemic.

I did a presentation to the National Association of Health Care Patient Advocates dealing with social isolation and how advocates can help. I also did an interview with Dr. Tony Gorceny, the chair of the Psychology Department at Chatham University in Pittsburgh.

In a McKnight Publication February 9, 2022 they cited a study: "Social isolation increases cardiovascular risk in older woman." The study of nearly 60,000 post-menopausal women found the risk of heart disease rose 27% of those who had limited social contact and felt isolated from others.

In the same article, The World Health Organization recognized social isolation and loneliness as a public health problem. According to the Centers of Disease Control and Prevention, being socially disconnected can increase the risk of death and increase the risk of dementia by 50%.

In another article in the *McKnight's Clinical Publication Daily*, February 17, 2022 titled, "Pandemic has eroded patient safety gains," researcher Amy Novotney argues that the COVID-19 pandemic significantly degraded the strides made over the last two decades in improving patient safety, particularly in long-term care.

An article, published in the *New England Journal of Medicine*, pointed to a "substantial deterioration" on multiple patient-safety metrics since the beginning of the pandemic. Healthcare-associated infections (HAIs), for example, increased significantly during 2020, reversing years of progress.

A PERSONAL PANDEMIC

My Personal Pandemic – "For Such A Time As This"

My name is Marla Turnbull and my Personal Pandemic began in January 2020. I slowly developed lower back pain as I continued through my rigorous work and family schedule. I was coming off of a challenging holiday work schedule, working long demanding days for a diamond distributor and a non-profit Foundation then heading into the new year caring for a very influential Pittsburgh Philanthropist and the additional 6 or so cases with Caregiver Champion. Speaking and leading my own business, Nature's Divine Healing, and serving as a member with NAIPC

(National Aging in Place Council) my body was deteriorating and I didn't realize it. At age 54, I was loving how I was helping others and making a difference in their lives.

My family had planned a 30th birthday party for my oldest daughter, Jenny, staying halfway to Charlotte, NC, where my youngest daughter, Laura, and her husband, Philip, lived. I did not want to miss this occasion. We booked an Air BNB at the New River Gorge in West Virginia where we would arrive on 2/28/2020 and stay all together for the weekend. We stayed 30 miles north of Beckley, West Virginia.

The weekend before our trip to the New River Gorge brought severe lower back pain and fatigue. I kept telling myself I was okay. I had pulled my lower back before and recovered. Why would this time be any different? This time the pain was excruciating. On Saturday, February 22, 2020, my oldest daughter, Jenny, drove me to a University of Pittsburgh Medical Center ER in the suburbs. I was chilled and had a slight fever. All I could do was lay under a cover shivering, after getting x-rays on my back. The pain was so bad I had to lay with my knees bent at a 90-degree angle. The resident came into my room and told me I had degenerative back disease and had to get this prescription of pain medicine filled. She stood at the foot of my bed and never touched or examined me. Never once asking for a urinalysis. She told me to follow up with an orthopedic doctor the next week.

On Wednesday, February 26, 2020, my daughter-in-law, Sarah, drove me to my orthopedic doctor's appointment. My mental decline was beginning to take a toll on me. The pain and fatigue were getting worse each day and sitting was difficult. The pain medicine and muscle relaxant were not taking the "edge" off. Again, more x-rays and a confirmed diagnosis of degenerative back disease. The doctor's orders were to go home, take the medications and rest. Again, no urinalysis was done.

I slept most of the next 2 days as we began packing for our weekend trip to W VA. I really did not want to miss my daughter's 30th birthday. On Friday, 2/28/2020, my husband, Steve, Jenny, and Sarah noticed increasing mental & body fatigue and confusion. They decided if I got "in trouble" there was a hospital in West Virginia close by where we were staying. I slept the entire 4-hour drive to our Air BNB. I do not remember much of anything after leaving Pittsburgh.

Once we arrived at our location, I remember being extremely exhausted and fatigued and needing a bed to lay down in. After resting a bit, I awoke and searched to find a bathroom. I tried looking for it but wound up in a closet. I called out to my husband for help. He came to help and said he needed to get me to the hospital ASAP. I put on my shoes and we made the 30-minute trip to Raleigh General Hospital in Beckley, West Virginia. Morgantown Hospital was an option, but it was 2 hours away. Time was of the essence so Beckley was the closest option.

Once I arrived at the ER, there were approximately 30 people waiting in line. I was triaged and sent immediately to the front of the line. The secretary in triage was worried about me and made the decision to have me seen ASAP.

It was determined through a urinalysis that I had a severe UTI from Staphylococcus Aurelia. The infection had moved into my blood stream. Additional tests were needed to determine the severity and areas that were under attack. My diagnosis was hard to immediately determine as the hospital used an off-site lab. The hospital personnel knew right away by looking at me that whatever I had was very critical. I still remember very little of these events.

The doctors began the barrage of testing on me. A spinal tap was done thinking I may have meningitis. Everyone who came near me wore extensive PPE covering. Additional tests included blood work, CT and MRI scans and a heart doppler. I was put on continuous oxygen and wore a pulse ox and full-leg air compressors on at all times. I had 5-6 IVs going, at least 3-5 antibiotics and fluids all at once. Walking to the "bathroom", a toilet next to my bed in the same room, was difficult. I need the help of 2 adults to sit me up in bed and walk me to the toilet 10 feet away.

I was in Septic Shock. The infection moved through my bloodstream straight to my heart. I developed a 1.7 cm bacterial growth on my mitral valve. The bacteria began to break off and travel to my left frontal cortex in my brain causing little mini strokes. I had infection in my neck, lower back, left psoas (hip) and right hip joint. I had nodules in both lungs and 1 kidney. A blood clot was found in my left hip as well.

From 9 pm on Friday, February 28th, 2020 through the next day, I was in a very deep sleep. I felt as if my body was floating through the room, often looking down on my situation. I can recollect being in a "library" floating around freely. There was a very gentle and friendly golden retriever by my side at all times. He followed me and stayed just beyond arm's reach. In this "library", I would look at the rows and rows of books on the shelves. One shelf appeared to hold the books of the Old Testament. I continue to be drawn to them. They were written in Hebrew, but I could read and understand the writings. Mind you, I have never read or spoken Hebrew. There was so much peace all around me and I was never afraid. The peace was so real I wanted to stay there forever. To this day, I still sense the peace in my heart and have no fear of death. This experience has truly brought me close to God in a very personal way.

I stayed in the ICU at Raleigh General Hospital for 7 days, staying an extra 2 days because I was waiting for a bed to become available in the ICU department at Presbyterian/Montefiore hospital. A very kind and seasoned nurse suggested we apply for a room on the regular floor, thinking my chances for transfer to Pittsburgh would be quicker. She was right, a bed did open up. There was a bed on the regular floor, which meant I had to be able to walk by myself to the bathroom. I worked on walking for the next 2 days and sure enough, I was able to navigate on my own.

The staff at Raleigh General Hospital was superb, skilled, and very professional. At the end of my stay at Raleigh General, the CEO asked to come to my room and visit me. He was very impressed by my quick recovery and the progress I was making. He was very kind and asked how he and his staff could continue providing high quality health care to the community. We had a wonderful discussion. He loved what he did, helping the sick get the care they needed. I told him how blessed I was to be at his hospital, for such a time as this. His staff was able to quickly diagnose and treat me; otherwise, I would not be alive today.

My daughter-in-law, Sarah was wonderful in keeping Jeff Weinberg at Caregiver Champion informed on my medical condition. He was instrumental in walking me through many aspects with my care. He would call weekly and check on me to make sure I was navigating through the myriad of medical decisions. One thing I remember Jeff saying was I had been through major trauma and it was going to take me awhile to recover. I needed to be patient and let my body heal. He said I was very fortunate to not have had more complications from the sepsis. At one point, my roommate was keeping me up at all hours of the night. He said I needed to ask the nurses to switch me to another room. I did not realize I could make the request. Once I did and my roommate was moved, I was able to get more sleep at night and heal much quicker.

Next, I was transported by ambulance to Presbyterian/Montefiore Hospital in Pittsburgh, PA. I was now ready to make the 4-hour trip to receive extended care closer to home. We left Raleigh General Hospital on Friday, March 6, 2020, at 8 pm. I arrived at midnight at an enormous and brightly lit hospital sitting high on a hill and sparkling in the distance. As I was being wheeled into the ER, I looked all around and saw the most beautiful castle, brightly illuminated with crystal chandeliers, marble floors and dark wooden doors. I truly felt like Esther in the Bible entering the King's palace.

We had heard that Covid-19 was making its way to the hospital and beds were being saved in advance of the projected onslaught of sick patients. Once the hospital Covid-19 protocol was in place, I was limited to one visitor per day. Once I arrived in my room, I headed straight to bed. I was in awe that I was now "home" and working toward greater recovery. A lengthy battery of tests was ordered for early Saturday and Sunday. CT and full-body MRI scans, x-rays of my neck and lower back, heart doppler and echocardiogram, vascular scan checking for blood clots on both of my groin areas and tons of blood work. I had doctors from every department assessing me: neurology, infectious disease, pulmonary, orthopedic and cardiology.

Since I had a previous blood clot, I would begin with a blood thinning medicine that would continue until the end of September.

Each day I would take several walks in my hospital hallway. My goal was to get out of bed and walk at least to the nurse's station about 20 yards down the hall. I soon realized, if I could make it to the nurse's station, I could go further each day. There were a couple motivators getting me out of bed. I knew if I could improve my walking, going farther each day, I would not have to meet with physical therapy. In addition, my lungs would get stronger so I didn't have to blow into the spirometry that measures your oxygen output. If I could not do those two things, I would walk each day until I was released. My goal was to walk a mile or more by the time of discharge. And, it worked!

The only thing holding me back, at this point, was getting my blood thinned so I could go on medication for the next six months before going home. Before being released, a nurse came to insert my PICC line. At home, I would be responsible to daily change my antibiotic bag and clean out my PICC line. A weekly visit from a home health nurse, PT and delivery of my home supplies was being arranged. Now I was getting anxious. The doctors remarked that they have never seen the miraculous healing from a Sepsis patient, as sick as I was. No surgeries were needed and everything healed by God's grace. Right before I was released after21 days in the hospital, I began taking my whole-food, plant-based capsules called Juice Plus. The vegetable, fruit and berry capsules contained whole food that the water and sugar were removed and the powder put into capsules. These capsules were my "miracle medicine" that kick started the healing process until eventually I was 100% healed.

Once at home, I wish I could say I was 100% healed, but the recovery was still far off. I began doing memory puzzles and brain games to regain my mental capacity. I required frequent naps during the day. Physical therapy visited my home and gave me weekly exercises to rebuild the muscle in my legs, arms, and abdomen. I daily worked on my balance and strength. The biggest hurdle was that friends and family expected me to act "normal" and pick up where I left off again since I was home. They didn't understand I was still healing. During this time we were in a lockdown so we had no visitors except nursing care. Each day I set a goal to get me through the mundane, day in and day out. Each day I picked one kitchen cabinet or drawer in the house to organize. I prided myself upon accomplishing this daily task.

I was home March through the beginning of August. My PICC line finally was finally removed in mid-June after getting clearance from the Infectious Disease doctor. Three more head to torso MRIs were done to determine if the infection had gone away in my neck and lower back. I do have to admit, after the devastating news the infection was still present after MRI #3 and #4, I questioned if I would ever be able to return to work. Finally in August 2020, after receiving the news that a much-improved MRI #5 showed the infection was GONE, I was slowly ready to go back to work.

Looking back, I realized there definitely was patient neglect initially in my care. By not ruling out a UTI initially, especially as a post-menopausal woman greater than 50 years old, was not standard of care. I did not file for medical malpractice for personal reasons and I am still torn on this issue.

The only person I know of who went through a greater missed diagnosis was my sister, Jeanie, who developed sepsis 2 years prior. She was released from a rural Ohio hospital too soon. The sepsis settled on her spinal cord in her neck. Five days after her release from the hospital, she could not walk or use her arms. She now was a quadriplegic and live 4 years before passing away in June

2021.Jeanie's second battle with sepsis, that led to her death, came after developing 2 bed sores in the nursing home that turned septic in June 2021. One of the nurses at the nursing home walked into her room at bedtime and found Jeanie unresponsive. This time, she had a heart attack after the sepsis traveled to her bones and one kidney. Once at the hospital, the doctors said it was too late to do surgery to remove the infected kidney. The day Jeanie was admitted after her heart attack, she signed a settlement winning a lawsuit for medical malpractice. Her dream was to be able to live on her own, with home care, using the money from her settlement. Once she realized the amount of money would not cover her entire home care for her remaining years, she gave up hope and immediately her health declined rapidly sending her to the hospital. She passed away several days later. The "cost of Covid-19" and the social isolation from being quarantined in her room alone, with no daily visits from my mom or her friends took a toll on Jeanie mentally.

She had survived Covid-19, but the social isolation was more than she could handle.

March 20, 2022, marks 2 years, to the date, since I came home from Presbyterian/Montefiore Hospital. What have I been up to? I have been able to continue life as I knew it before sepsis. I work for my own company, Natures Divine Healing, LLC as a Master Certified Health & Wellness Coach. For the last year, I went back to school and graduated with a Master's degree. In October 2022, I will sit for Boards to become a National Board-Certified Health & Wellness Coach. I like to say that I get paid to change the genetics/DNA of those I work with and future generations. Going back to school really challenged me to pivot to the next level and work on getting my memory back. I knew I had to really take time to study, read and memorize during this past year. I am in awe as I truly did not know if I could reach this milestone. I am happy to report, I graduated as one of the Valedictorians in my class.

Today, I am being asked to speak and share my testimony and health and wellness with senior groups. Social isolation, shame from "not being enough" to family members during the Pandemic, and daily chronic stress are what I spend the majority of my time helping my clients overcome. In addition, I work with Corporations on Health, Wellness, Chronic Stress and Employee Retention as the Covid-19 pandemic has taken our society from the "Great Resignation" to the "Great Upgrade". I was asked to be on the University of Pittsburgh Stakeholder Advisory Board for Sepsis and Pneumonia in June 2020. I continue as a member of the Greater Pittsburgh National Aging in Place Council and I am a member of the United Way of Southwestern Pennsylvania Women's Leadership Council. I absolutely love what I do and cannot imagine doing anything different. My Personal pandemic was the perfect timing "For such a time as this".

—Marla Turnbull
Master Certified Health & Wellness Coach

You can see an interview with Marla on YouTube Caregiver Champion.

What Are The Solutions?

Issues and problems have been stated throughout this book—how can they be fixed.

One way is by having family members, trusted friends or paid professionals advocate by looking out for you or your loved one in a complex, fragmented system.

Patient Advocates can help individuals, but it does not change the system.

So what else can help?

There are some new models of care from professionals who have created a new way of thinking about nursing homes and resident care.

Patient-Centered Care

As described throughout this book, the care provided in hospitals and nursing homes is largely impersonal today. Impersonal care is hardly care at all. One of the reasons I love to work with the elderly is getting to know their history, their childhood, their occupation, their families. I have always felt that I have been enriched learning about people's lives. A colleague who has helped edit this book, Ann Gatey, had a pet therapy dog that would go into residents' rooms and visit once a week. She knew more about the residents than the staff, because she took the time to listen while they were petting her dog.

When I teach administration, on the first day of class I pass out this poem called "See Me":

See Me

What do you see, nurses, what do you see?
Are you thinking, when you look at me —
A crabby old woman, not very wise,
Uncertain of habit, with far-away eyes,
Who dribbles her food and makes no reply,
When you say in a loud voice — "I do wish
    you'd try."

Who seems not to notice the things that
    you do,
And forever is losing a stocking or shoe,
Who unresisting or not, lets you do as
    you will,
With bathing and feeding, the long day to fill.
Is that what you're thinking, is that what
    you see?
Then open your eyes, nurse, you're looking
    at ME...
I'll tell you who I am, as I sit here so still;
As I rise at your bidding, as I eat at your will.

I'm a small child of ten with a father
    and mother,
Brothers and sisters, who love one another,
A young girl of sixteen with wings on her feet.
Dreaming that soon now a lover she'll meet;
A bride soon at twenty — my heart gives
    a leap,
Remembering the vows that I promised
    to keep;
At twenty-five now I have young of my own,
Who need me to build a secure, happy home;
A woman of thirty, my young now grow fast,
Bound to each other with ties that should last;
At forty, my young sons have grown and
    are gone,
But my man's beside me to see I don't mourn;
At fifty once more babies play 'round my knee,
Again we know children, my loved one
    and me.

Dark days are upon me, my husband is dead,
I look at the future, I shudder with dread,
For my young are all rearing young of
    their own,
And I think of the years and the love that
    I've known;
I'm an old woman now and nature is cruel —

'Tis her jest to make old age look like a fool.
The body is crumbled, grace and vigor depart,
There is now a stone where once I had a heart,
But inside this old carcass a young girl
    still dwells,
    And now and again my battered
    heart swells.

I remember the joys, I remember the pain,
And I'm loving and living life over again,
I think of the years, all too few —
    gone too fast,
And accept the stark fact that nothing
    can last —
So I open your eyes, nurses, open and see,
Not a crabby old woman, look closer, nurses —
    see ME!

This poem was found among the possessions of an elderly lady who died in the geriatric ward of a hospital. No information is available concerning her — who she was or when she died. Reprinted from the "Assessment and Alternatives Help Guide" prepared by the Colorado Foundation for Medical Care.

I once had a client who has since passed away, who was an attorney and was part of a lawsuit against the NFL for causing concussions in football players. Another client had gone through the Holocaust, another owned a dairy farm, and another was a Rabbi and a psychologist.

Once you find out these facts about the person, it's hard to call the person the hip or knee in room 232!

The National Alliance for Mental Illness (NAMI) has a saying, "See the PERSON and Not The CONDITION. Take the pledge." Everyone in health care needs to take the pledge! www.nami.org/stigmafree

I had a client who had a terrible automobile accident and was taken to a hospital called Mercy Hospital. It used to be run by the Sisters of Mercy. He became a quadriplegic. From the first day he was admitted they kept telling his wife, he wasn't going to live, even though each day he was progressing and recovering. When he was admitted a social worker asked his wife, "What are your expectations?" She told her she wanted him to recover and go back to work in a limited capacity. The social worker told her that there was no way this could happen. I was called to help this family and I met with the treatment team and the patient and his wife. I began by asking them, since they were taken over by a non-religious hospital, did the caring and the mercy stop?

I told them that their lives had been turned around on a dime, yet no one was giving them the emotional support to help them. It was easier to get them out of the hospital so they could get another "Head in the Bed".

Today, my client does need total care. But he is in a motorized wheelchair which he can use independently. His company bought him a computer he can use that is voice activated.

And he is able to drive a van!

I once provided an Inservice to Activities Professionals for CEU's called "Activities is more than playing bingo." My mother-in-law hated bingo so when they played 4 or 5 times a week, she would sit at the nurse's station doing nothing. Meanwhile she loved music, she was an accomplished pianist, and conducted musicals at her condominium in Florida. She also enjoyed reading and interacting with others. No one bothered to find out her interests and foster them.

The Thrive Model

This model moves away from the medical model and adds to the patient center care model. The philosophy is to engage your residents to Thrive not Survive. Anna Freud actually developed this model for children and their mental health. The focus is on well-being.

The Prevention Institute vision is that all people experience their full potential for health, safety, and well-being across the country through these principles:

- **Belonging and creating** a vision that all people experience their full potential for health, safety, and well-being; having a place, feeling part of something

- **Safety:** the experience of security and stability at the interpersonal, emotional, and community level

- **Dignity:** the experience of having worth/value; living in a climate of mutual respect and regard

- **Trust:** the ability to rely on the wider community, government, and public institutions

- **Hope and aspiration:** the belief that progress is possible

- **Control of destiny and self-determination:** the ability to take action and lead change

The Eden Alternative

One of my most admired leaders in the aging field is Dr. Bill Thomas.

Dr. Thomas was an ER physician and was asked to be a medical director at a nursing home. Once there, he knew the model had to change. He said, no one grows up with the goal that their aging years should end in a nursing home. (YouTube Dr. Bill Thomas: https://www.youtube.com/watch). Dr. Thomas felt that residents were **largely lonely, helpless and bored.**

With that in mind he created the Eden Alternative.

The guiding principles of the Eden Alternatives are called DOMAINS OF WELL-BEING ™.

IDENTITY- Being well-known; having personhood; individuality; wholeness; having a history

GROWTH- Development; enrichment; unfolding, expanding; evolving

AUTONOMY- Liberty; self-governance; self-determination; immunity from the arbitrary exercise of authority; choice; freedom

SECURITY- Freedom from doubt; anxiety; fear; assured; having privacy; dignity, and respect

CONNECTIVENESS- State of being connected; alive; belonging; engaged; involved; not detached; connected to the past, present, and the future; connected to personal possessions; connected to place; connected to nature

MEANING- Significance; heart; hope; import; value; purpose; reflection; sacred

JOY- Happiness; pleasure; delight; contentment; enjoyment

These domains are the guiding principles of the Eden Alternative.

There are about 300 nursing homes in the United States and some in Australia and in Europe. (Please go to YouTube and check out The Eden Alternative Experience: https://www.youtube.com/watch?v=qK3vTbckZMw) It will make you smile and make your heart feel good.

I always say that I can evaluate how good a nursing home is in 5 minutes after walking into the facility because it has a pulse!

This means there is positive interaction, laughter between the residents and the staff. Residents are not sitting at the nurse's station or the tv room just staring.

The other important factor is that the staff are called Care Partners. Everyone's responsibility is to take care of all of the residents.

I was once an interim administrator in a facility and on my first day I was walking the hall (which I did every day) and someone rang their call bell and said she had to go to the bathroom. Two nursing assistants were walking down the hall and I told them the resident needed to go to the bathroom. One nursing assistant told me that she was not assigned to the room and continued walking. The other told me she was going to lunch and kept walking, at which point, I stopped them and told them they both could keep walking out the door!

This made the staff learn in a hurry that it was everybody's responsibility to answer call bells.

The Green House Model

Dr. Bill Thomas created this model to truly change a nursing home from a medical model to a true home model. These are smaller structures housing just 10-12 residents with dedicated staff. (Please check out The Green House Project: Revolutioning Care)

Dr Bill Thomas felt hat there needed to be a person in long term care who protected, sustained and nurtured the elderly. He found a Persian legend about a royal falcon who watched over the kingdom... this is the **Shabazim**, the versatile worker within The Green House model.

This is truly exciting https://www.youtube.com/channel/UC5RU2lqtlrZ5yoTj_RID1dg

In an AARP article entitled "Lessons from the Green House Staffing Model" dated February 4, 2022; A national evaluation of the Green House Model demonstrated that the Green House homes consistently performed in the top tier of nursing homes on clinical /health outcomes of residents, with fewer incidents of Covid 19 and deaths.

The program was funded by the Robert Wood Johnson Foundation, (A Foundation that usually funds innovative projects for seniors).

To date, more than 260 Green House homes in 32 states are open or under development. And in general, studies suggest that elders living in the homes are happier and healthier. For more information check out https://thegreenhouseproject.org/resources/research/

The bad news is that these facilities are very costly. A facility in Pennsylvania called Londonderry advertises their rate as $435/day. This is approximately twice the rate of a typical assisted living facility. There is no government funding. Hopefully someday there will be funding by raising awareness of this amazing program.

This hasn't stopped Dr. Thomas from continuing to improve for the aged.

In 2014, Dr. Thomas collaborated with Kavan Peterson, to create the Changing Aging Tour. The Changing Aging Tour directly addressed damaging myths about aging and featured two non-fiction theater performances in a "pro-aging festival." Over the next four years this tour performed in over 130 cities across North America. Also in 2014, Dr Thomas contributed to developing a Geriatric ER in hospitals. This was taken on by the Geriatric Development Collaborative (GEDC), which is dedicated to the optimal emergency care of older adults.

GEDC is a nationwide collaborative dedicated to improving the quality of care for older people in Emergency Departments with the goal of reducing harm and improving health care outcomes. They are committed to making change through the education of individuals, and hospital-wide initiatives that create sustainable improvements in practice at all levels.

The Milken Institute: The Center For Future Aging

Although it appears that Dr. Bill Thomas is the only person trying to advance aging services, there are others including the Milken Institute.

The Milken Institute is a nonprofit, nonpartisan think tank that helps people build meaningful lives, in which they can experience health and well-being. They have been exploring Long Term Care Services and Dementia Care and funding resources.

In June 2021, the Institute established a round table discussion with leaders in the field across the country to explore ways to improve and pay for comprehensive dementia care.

Action steps included :

1. Ensure all dementia care models contain minimum set of core elements for comprehensive care
2. Implement quality care models to develop outcomes of these models
3. Expand dementia-specific training
4. Test implementation of payment models
5. Develop mechanism to pay community-based organizations

To read the full report visit:
milkeninstitute.org/report/
dementia-care-models-scalling:comprehensive

Architecture firms are developing new concepts for nursing homes where residents would live in pods so they could develop immunity and be isolated from infectious diseases from the facility.

All of these are wonderful and innovative concepts that would surely improve nursing home care but there is still huge stumbling blocks the government and pharmaceuticals.

CONGRESS AND THEIR BENEFITS

The Indeed Editorial Team in February 2021 highlighted Congress and their benefits:

Congressmen and senators purchase their insurance through an Affordable Care Act exchange. 72% of their premiums are covered by a federal subsidy. When they retire, they can qualify for lifetime health insurance under the Federal Employees Health Benefits Program.

After serving for five years, a member of Congress is eligible for a pension. Their retirement benefits depend on their plan, age and how long they served in Congress. A member of Congress can collect their full pension at the age of 62 or if they are age 50 with 20 years of service. Though it is a common belief that they can earn their full salary amount in retirement, this is not true. They can earn up to 80% of their final salary. The salary on the average is $174,000 per year.

If a member of Congress dies while serving in office, their family can receive a payout equivalent to a year's salary.

> Every member of Congress has paid into Social Security since 1984. They are eligible for the same Social Security benefits as all other participants. Likewise, members of Congress who have been elected after 1984 also pay into and are covered by the Federal Employees Retirement System (FERS). After five years of full participation, they become vested.

So to summarize, Congress has no incentive to increase benefits for Medicare, Social Security and Medicaid.

Statista Research Department, recently published that, a little more than 54 percent of Americans had an annual household income that was less than 75,000 U.S. dollars.

This is 50% less than what Congress gets at $174,000

Although they do get Social Security, after 5 years of service they are eligible at 62 for 80% of their full salary.

Their Health Insurance is subsidized at 72% of their premium and when they retire, they qualify for lifetime health benefits through Federal Employees Health Benefits Program.

Did anybody hear anything about MEDICARE AND MEDICAID, I DIDN'T!

I always say, put Congress on an equal playing field and they then would pay attention to what the average American needs when they age and retire!

According to the Federal Budget, in 2019, major entitlement programs-Social Security, Medicare, Medicaid, Obamacare, and other health care programs-consumed 51 percent of all federal spending, larger than the portion of spending for other national priorities (such as national defense) combined.

Almost every year Congress tries to cut or eliminate one of these benefits.

So it appears we know what to do based on some of the pioneers, like Dr. Bill Thomas, and The Milken Institute and others. However, we have little interest by Congress to fund and change the programs.

We have gone full circle back to the beginning of the book. The care in healthcare and long-term care has largely gone away. We have a moral and ethical dilemma. Should everybody have the right to have access to healthcare, affordable prescriptions and proper long-term care? In the United States the answer is a resounding NO. In other countries this is not the case. They may pay higher taxes but they are able to provide healthcare for all, with every nationality having equal access to care. Their morbidity and mortality rate are actually higher than the USA and there appears to be a cultural belief that the elderly are not a burden but a valuable member of society and should be treated with the dignity and respect they deserve.

In conclusion, this book has attempted to explain how the healthcare system works or in many instances doesn't work;. It has provided an overview or primer that helps the reader understand how systems are reimbursed.

It has discussed Medicare, Medicaid and Obama Care benefits and Innovative alternatives to care. So what next?

Advocacy, Advocacy, And Advocacy

1. Contact your congressman anytime you feel there is something being proposed that can help improve care or stop a bill from being passed if it is going to reduce care or benefits.

2. Join AARP, the American Association of Retired Persons. They are more than a place that you can get seniors' discount. They have an entire division that works to lobby for improvement of healthcare and benefits.

3. Join specific organizations like the Alzheimer's Association.

4. Attend lectures and read articles and books on areas of health care that interest you.

5. Contact the Ombudsman or the Department of Health if your loved one is not getting the care they need and deserve.

6. Hire a Health Care Patient Advocate to help you navigate the Health Care Maze and get the care you need and deserve.

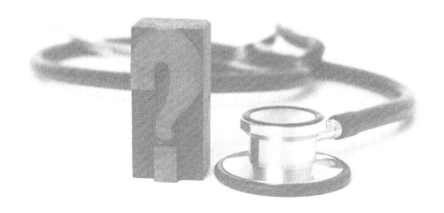

RESOURCES

This last section will provide you with resources to use to help you navigate this broken healthcare maze.

A. The Josie King Foundation

In February, 2001 Josie King an 18-month infant died of a medical error inn the hospital.

Since then her mother Sorrel King has dedicated her life to help prevent medical errors from occurring in the hospital. Her mother wrote a book, *Josie's Story*, that documents the medical error, the families' emotions and ultimately establishing the Foundation.

For a nominal fee one can purchase the Care Journal or download an app that helps you navigate the hospital healthcare maze and helps you remember conversations with nurses and physicians. Prepare questions to ask; and even where you parked!

B. The Care Partner Project (CarePartnerProject.org}

Developed Hospital Stay Checklists as a result of its founder, Karen Curtis, almost dying of sepsis while in the hospital.

A colleague of mine was seen in the emergency room and was misdiagnosed and almost died from Sepsis which then spread to every organ in her body. I did a You tube video with her titled The Silent UTI which Everyone Needs to Know https://www.youtube.com/watch?v=yaoqRPIingA

The Care Partner Project developed extensive checklists for Emergency Room Visits and Hospital Stay.

A few of them include:

- SuperBug Infections (Staph, MRSA, VRE) main issue is Handwashing, following infection control procedures and room cleaning.

- Sepsis
- Medication Mistakes- Nurse should identify patient by asking for a birthdate, tell the patient what is being given and stay there while the pill is given so she watches for choking or side effects
- How to prevent Bed Sores (Nurse should check skin every day and patient should be turned and repositioned every 2 hours.

C. The Greater National Advocates

Developed by L. Bradley Schwartz, who is an attorney and lost all of his limbs due to medical errors.

He is now dedicated to helping caregivers. He has an advocate directory listing anyone in the country who is a patient advocate (I'm in it).

He provides training for anyone who wants to learn to be a patient advocate. I also interviewed Bradley, it is a You Tube Video under Caregiver Champion https://www.youtube.com/channel/UC X4jfZWtrM4-rUAn5xW0SCg

D. The Pa. Health and Wellness (Pa. Health and Wellness.com)

Published an article called "Are You Ready to See the Doctor?"

The average doctor spends 7 minutes with their patients and probably less while in the hospital. They usually make rounds at 5am or 9pm

A client of mine was told she was not allowed to visit until 10 am because the doctor and his team made rounds before that!

I told them that was the very reason why she should be allowed to visit, and got that changed.

On another occasion, a physiatrist, (doctor of rehab medicine) denied sending my client's mother to a rehab hospital after being in the hospital. When I asked why the doctor denied her, I was told she is the chief of physiatry and that was her decision! I asked her to talk with me and the patient's daughter about what was the basis of her decision and she refused. This now had become a Patient Rights issue as people are entitled to find out and know about their care. I reported her to the medical director and the patient representative of the hospital.

So you can see why it is important to be organized and prepared when you are seeing a doctor.

The article suggests the following:

1. **Get organized before your appointment**

   Make a list of questions starting with the most important

   Report any changes of condition since last appointment

   Bring a list of medications and make sure you understand what and why you are taking them

2. **During your appointment**

   Be specific about your symptoms and problems

   Review your list of questions

   Take notes

   Bring a friend or relative to the appointment (Caregiver Champion provides a nurse to go to appointments when a family member cannot)

   Schedule your next appointment, labs, or tests before you leave the office

3. **After your appointment review your notes and instructions**

   Pick up any prescriptions at the pharmacy (Do not use old medications that have been discontinued) A majority of hospital-izations and rehospitalizations are caused by not following the physician's instructions and not taking the medication prescribed

4. Complete lab or diagnostic tests

What to look for when choosing a nursing home or personal care home

1. When you get a list of nursing homes from the hospital, call people you know to see if they know someone in that facility and what was their experience (Caregiver Champion vets nursing facilities so we can give you the top three in your area.)

2. Visit the facility unannounced (usually after 5pm after the administrative staff have left.) Then if you like it ask for a tour the next day

3. Ask to see their last nursing home survey. They are usually in a public place in the lobby

4. The Federal Government through cms.gov / nursinghomecompare can provide you the rating of any nursing facility in the country.

This rating is based on a 5-star rating system including nursing home surveys, deficiencies, quality standards and complaints.

5. As discussed before check how the staff interacts with the residents, and how they interact with each other. Is the facility active or lifeless with residents sitting at the nursing station staring or are they engaged with the staff?

6. All of the traits that Dr. Bill Thomas spoke about are the very things you are looking for in a nursing facility.

7. If the person is going for rehab and then going home, do they have a separate area for rehab patients or are they mixed with the resident population. Most Rehab patients do not want to be mixed with long term stay residents.

8. Is the nursing home currently at full staffing levels for nurses, aids and other workers? If they are working short staff or with a lot of agency staff, your loved one will probably not get the type of care needed.

9. How is the facility handling Covid-19?

10. Have there been Covid outbreaks in the last two weeks?

11. How does the facility currently handle visitation?

12. How is the facility communicating important Covid-19 information?

13. How does the facility allow virtual communication?

14. **DO NOT ALLOW** the hospital to send your family member to a nursing home that you have not approved of!

Why Should You Use a Health Care Patient Advocate?

This book has shown that the Emperor Does Need New Clothes!

In order to improve health care, we need to have a major culture change.

This change requires that all Americans should have access to health care, no matter of race, creed, color or national origin. Americans should be able to afford their medications. We should be providing person centered care. Caring about the person should be most important not bottom-line profits. Nursing homes should be treating the resident with the dignity and respect they deserve, not just paying lip service to those words.

However, this will not occur in my lifetime. We have politics, pharmaceuticals, health insurance policies all preventing this cultural change.

As a result, anyone trying to navigate the health care maze and doesn't have someone knowledgeable about health care should hire an advocate. Hospitals, Nursing homes, Home Health Care all have someone who is called a patient advocate, but they are working for the facility and not you!

1. A health care patient advocate works as a partner with you and represents you.

2. They understand the healthcare system and how it is reimbursed.

3. They help you ask questions that you might not have thought of so that you may have a better understanding and learn about alternatives so that you can make intelligent choices.

4. They help you understand your health coverage and understand medical bills that you receive.

5. They are experts in Disease Management or they find someone who is.

6. They help with Medication Management.

7. If you live out of town, they provide you some comfort and relief knowing that your loved one's care is being managed

   I call this "Boots on the Ground" as we become the eyes and ears for the relative living out of town.

8. They say "No" to authorities that are making you do or choose something that is not in the best interest of the patient. I give a class on "you can say no to a discharge social worker." So you don't allow someone to send your loved one to a facility that you have not vetted or they want to discharge prematurely and the patient is acutely ill.

   I was once called on a Sunday during a Steeler Football game from a client whose mother was being discharged on a Sunday. I drove to the facility and stopped the discharge. They insisted they had informed the mother of the discharge, however the mother did not understand what that meant and the family was not prepared for her to come home so it was an unsafe discharge. I actually spoke to a regional supervisor who lived across the state and he finally cancelled the discharge.

9. Patient advocates make sure the person care is quality and meets the standard for someone's care in the hospital or nursing home. They advocate for you by meeting with doctors ,nurses, rehab professionals, the interdisciplinary team and attend care conferences when care is not being given properly and try to work out a plan that is in the best interest for the client or patient.

10. They assure that your rights as a patient and an individual are being followed and protected.

My website has a lot more information about Health Care Patient Advocacy. caregiverchampionadvocate.com. It also has video interviews that we did on various topics including advocacy.

We interviewed a pioneer in the field on advocacy Ann Llewyn and it can be seen at https://www.facebook.com/CaregiverChampionAdvocates/videos/1164223200624815/ Please check it out.

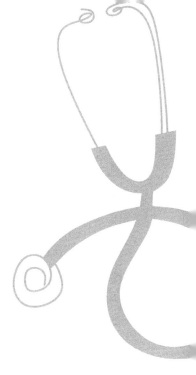

Conclusion

This concludes this book. I hope you can find it to be a useful tool as you take your journey through the healthcare maze. We have examined how the system is broken and provided you with some useful tools to cope with it. I have provided you with information about health insurance, Medicare and Medicaid. You have received information about useful resources that can help guide you on your journey as well as tools you can put in your toolbox, I hope that this will help you receive the quality care and caring that you and your family deserves. May your journey be safe and successful.

Personal Testimonials And My Services As A Health Care Patient Advocate

If you have ever tried to navigate the U S health system, you will know it's a nightmare. I had this experience last year in 2021. It was during Covid lockdown, plus I live over 3000 miles away in England. I attempted to deal with everything independently. It didn't take long for the feeling of desperation to set in. I realized I needed help. The Jewish Family Federation of Pittsburgh steered me to an advocate. I hired Jeff Weinberg, a skilled health care advocate. He was on the job immediately. Thanks to the technology of today, we managed to work together even though we were such a big distance apart. Jeff was a guardian angel to me and my brother (who died in peace). He went way beyond the call of duty and for this I'm eternally grateful. He was worth every penny and more. I know I could not have made my brothers last few weeks in life as comfortable and high quality without him.

—Dee Bellarby

—✳—o🏵o—✳—

What does 'care' mean in the context of being a 'care'-giver or a 'care'-manager for a person who is ascending into the depths of dementia?

On a high level, it means conceiving and executing a plan of meeting the needs of a startled, lost, mentally impaired individual. To provide proper 'care'/'caring' requires:

- an understanding of the individual in the context of their multi-dimensional personal history
- an understanding of their illness both broadly and specifically, its course, and how it has affected the individual's needs from 'baseline'
- an understanding of the individual's available support: amount of useable resources, the group of folks (and their respective baggage) with whom you will perform intensive teamwork as partners-in-'caring'
- a thorough, professional, and experienced understanding of the local medical, social,

residential, recreational, legal, political, and administrative landscape for 'caring'

- an understanding of how to cobble together intelligently, creatively, and productively a 'plan-of-care' that fits all the above to optimally meet a continually evolving (sometimes gradually, sometimes suddenly) constellation of needs

This planner/deliverer of customized 'care' is a person or persons with extreme empathy, patience, persistence, and wisdom; undaunted optimism, will, faith, and love. They must be honest, ethical, practical, as well as instinctively pay attention to and know where to look for details.

How do I know this? I was blessed to find Jeff Weinberg about 3 years ago when my brother crossed the threshold into needing a 'care'-plan and planner for his burgeoning dementia. Jeff has been teaching me the meaning of 'caring' ever since. He personifies 'care'-giving and 'caring'.

After a first meeting with Jeff, I emailed him to confirm that I needed his assistance. Based on my initial impressions, I wrote: "You can do more than assist—you can give my brother hope and dignity."

I have been correct since Day 1, and I continue to learn true meanings of 'caring', 'hope', 'dignity', and 'love' from Jeff along the way.

I can be reached at
jeff@caregiverchampionadvocate.com
or my website caregiverchampionadvocate.com

Best wishes

Jeff Weinberg, M.PH. M. Ed, NHA
Nationally Certified Health Care Patient Advocate

WA

Made in the USA
Coppell, TX
14 December 2022